The
Vodka
Diet
Protocol

> **"**
> An evidence-based protocol utilizing
> hormones, peptides, and nutrition.
>
> Yes! You can get into the shape of
> your life and have your martini too!
> **"**

Joseph Pace, MD
Cardiac Electrophysiologist

Thank you!

To my wife, Michele LeMay, MD
You have been an inspiration, my rock and guiding light!

To all my patients and to one, Chris Bogle
For your contribution here and continued success with the VDP

Please visit us on social media:
TheVodkaDiet.com
Instagram: TheVodkaDietGuy
YouTube: TheVodkaDiet
Facebook: TheVodkaDietPage

The Vodka Diet
Volume 1

Table of Contents

chapter

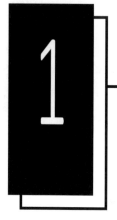

Introduction

H ello, Dr. Joseph Pace here! First, a big thank you for reading my book! Let me start by answering your first big question. Is there really a vodka diet? So, I can just drink vodka and get into the best shape of my life? Well, there is a lot more to it than that. The short answer is No. If you are looking for a quick fix, this may not be the protocol for you. This is an evidence-based, physician-supervised protocol utilizing hormones, peptides, nutrition, and fitness. Just so happens if you have your martini in the evening, you can have success!

Let me tell you a short story of how this came about. I am a cardiac electrophysiologist in a small town in Florida. I have spent my wonderful career putting in pacemakers, doing cardiac procedures, and treating heart disease. All the while in the back of my head I felt like we were missing something in medicine. I would have questions in my mind, such as, if statins are a multi-billion-dollar drug then why is heart disease the number one killer? Also, if thyroid medicine is the number one class of drugs, then why do so many of my patients feel so bad on it? Then I started looking into the field of nutrition and asked myself why do doctors get zero hours of nutrition in their many years of training? I just felt that there must be a better way. Where did medicine go wrong? Are we doing the best for our patients? Then I was introduced to the field of hormones or bio-identical hormone replacement therapy, BHRT. This field, along with peptides has opened my eyes to a new reality in medicine, and thus the purpose of this book.

So back to the vodka diet story. I have a patient, Chris Bogle that has done quite well utilizing the concepts laid out in what we call the vodka diet protocol or VDP. Chris originally was clinically obese with cholesterol numbers, blood pressure, diet, etc. all out of whack. He was heading down the heart attack trail. Come to think of it, the typical American. So, we started a protocol laid out in this book and Chris started to have some good results. While reviewing his labs one day we were talking about what was working etc. He admitted that during the protocol, he had a martini or two along the way thus, the birth of the VDP. Since then Chris and I have become friends, he is an industry professional in medicine, and we have learned a lot from each other.

With that being said, I have asked Chris to do some heavy lifting in this book as he has lived and experienced everything I have laid out in this book. What better way than to hear from someone that has lived it rather than reading some research or marketing brochure.

I have decided to present the VDP in more of a dialogue between a patient and a doctor. There are many areas in this book that have different opinions such as many areas of medicine. We lay this out in a way that you can see the different views. Chris and I will debate, agree, and agree to disagree in some areas for the purpose of you getting a 360-degree view and not one biased opinion. I will keep this at the patient level yet enlightening for the practitioners out there as well. We will have fun, hopefully, you will be entertained, educated, enlightened, and inspired to make some changes in your life.

Nothing in this book is meant to replace the advice of your physician.

A quick note to my physician colleagues out there. Hopefully, this book will help your patients seek out a pathway to healthcare, not sick care. My desire is to increase patients in your office seeking this protocol, not to increase patients in my office. Quite frankly the Cath lab keeps me very busy. In this book, purposely, there will be no brand names mentioned, so as not to be an infomercial. We have a website, YouTube, and Instagram for patients if they want to seek therapy in their area.

What's going to happen from here on out, Chris and I will share the microphone if you will. Again, Chris has lived this, has had great results and has done extensive research into these areas. Chris and I have also tapped into a panel of experts in different areas to bring you, the reader, a true 360 perspective into this.

Who is the VDP audience? A wide range of people: most likely the largest audience will be a range of men and women over 35 years of age. I say range because you can have hormone imbalances and the inability to lose fat and gain muscle at any age. The best way to find out if this book is for you is to ask yourself how you feel, and are you having trouble losing fat. If you are not feeling your best and you just know that something is not right, chances are good that your hormones are not optimized. Perhaps you are an MD, DO, ARNP, PA, RN looking at this from a clinical perspective. If that is the case, I have included some medium level clinical pearls, but most of this book is for the people. Also, you may be a thought leader in any of these areas, if so, please reach out as I would like to share the stage with you. Speaking of that, I have included the writings of some thought leaders in this volume and I am seeking more contributing authors in Volume two. Now a few words from my patient before we get started:

Hello! Thank you, Dr. Pace! Chris Bogle here. What an honor to share these pages with you! This has been an amazing journey, what an honor to share this with our readers as well! The purpose here is to describe an evidence-based protocol that has been proven by myself and others to change your body composition and introduce a new way of living. This book basically encompasses many different algorithms which are detailed herein.

So why the vodka diet you ask? Dr. Pace started the story above, and if you're like me, when five o'clock rolls around, you like to have your toddy. Does that ring a bell in your life? If so, you are not alone my friend! It is a well-known fact that once the body is processing alcohol, it stops processing fat. Well, Dr. Pace is about to lay out a plan that can circumvent that and work around your body's defenses and allow you to lose fat while gaining muscle. Second, I want to say I am not a medical doctor, a nurse, or a brilliant scientist.

My original career was as a chef in Texas, then I had a good run with big pharma for thirteen years. During those thirteen years, I learned so much about medicine, mostly in men's and women's health, with a concentration in hormone replacement therapy. I thought the way to live healthier was to stay sick and stay alive. Well I've learned there's so much more out there, and I'm so glad to share some of my learnings here with Dr. Pace. There is so much outside of the pharmaceutical world that can help you to live a healthier, leaner, happier life. I am not an expert; I have just lived the VDP lifestyle for a little over a year and have personally dove into the research presented here by Dr. Pace.

I wish I could express in words what a joy it is to achieve weight loss goals, and have the opportunity to share this information with you. So why am I joining Dr. Pace here? Quite simply, very few people know that bioidentical hormone replacement (BHRT) exists, and even fewer know about peptides. I have searched for a book or manuscript on this and could not find one. There is so much information out there of the individual topics, but not a plan, so now Dr. Pace lays out a plan for you in this book. Again, what an honor!

Hormones

2

D r. Pace here. Bio-Identical Hormone Replacement Therapy Pellets or "BHRT" has changed my life personally, as well as professionally. The bottom line is I feel great! BHRT will be the foundation and the future of this entire program. Think of hormones as the canvas, and the rest of the information as the artwork that'll be laid upon the canvas. Think of hormones as the universe, and everything else in this book as the solar systems in that universe. Think of hormones as the master. Think of hormones as the conductor. Think of hormones as the puppeteer, and everything else merely the puppets. For my spiritual friends - hormones - the omniscient - unlimited knowledge and omnipresent in all things. OK - So you get the point. This is the most important aspect of the entire program. I can't reiterate that enough.

When we talk about BHRT, exactly are we talking about? Let's take the big four: testosterone, estrogen, progesterone, and thyroid.

Testosterone

Think of this as the mother hormone, the master of them all, the ruler of the universe, the chosen one. First, let's get started with a big myth or misconception that many people have about testosterone. Do women have testosterone? Absolutely! We all know men have testosterone, and more on estrogen in men later. Humans cannot live without testosterone. With that being said let's just talk about women first, because you probably thought I was going to talk about men mostly in this section. Testosterone has an absolute profound impact on women, and it is amazing how it can change their life. Let's look at the big things that women present and complain about as they reach peri and post-menopause. Things such as libido, sleep, mood, depression, or energy to name a few. Any of that ring a bell? The only big thing that we want to differentiate here with women is night sweats and hot flashes as they are different things entirely. Testosterone will have a big impact on night sweats. That might be the first thing that will go away when you start on testosterone therapy. Hot flashes, on the other hand, you feel in the middle of your chest, and it's like a raging fire that goes all the way up to your head. These hot flashes will be subsided with estrogen. (More on estrogen later.)

Let's switch gears to men. Can we talk about erectile dysfunction here, or should we talk about all-cause mortality being increased in men with testosterone under a blood level of six hundred? In this book, we will talk about reference ranges on labs, and I will probably bring it up a time or two again. This is a good time to have a small discussion on reference ranges. If you were to go to a garden-variety primary care physician, nothing wrong with them, and let's say you're a fifty-year-old man. I'll use all-round numbers here. You may have a testosterone level of five hundred. On the reference ranges that might be on the high side of normal, with most labs. That primary care physician is going to say that you are normal, and more than likely would not prescribe testosterone therapy to you. Meanwhile, you have very little erectile function, you need a nap every day at three o'clock, the last time you saw the inside of a gym was when you paid for the membership and never returned. Get the point? In the VDP, we want your testosterone to be over one thousand for men, and a nice range for women is going to be one-hundred and fifty to three hundred. Once men get testosterone pellets, they can get into the eleven, twelve, thirteen-hundred range. Chris runs in the 1300 range.

Ladies if you get the three to four hundred don't be alarmed either, as there is no harm, and trust me, you will feel amazing. In addition to testosterone giving you such a great feeling, there are also many more benefits to testosterone that you cannot feel. Benefits to the heart, breast, bones, and brain that we refer to as asymptomatic benefits for men and women.

In order to break this down a little bit, let's start with women and their breasts. I know you may fear hormones because you think they will cause breast cancer. Early results from a study suggest that testosterone implanted under the skin as a pellet about every 3 months helped ease menopausal symptoms without raising a woman's risk of breast cancer. This is exactly what we do in my clinic and the VDP clinics around the country. The only difference here is that many women can go 3-5 months between pellet insertions. Also, in women, the enzyme aromatase converts some testosterone to estradiol, a type of estrogen. Because HRT has been found to increase breast cancer risk, doctors believe that estradiol converted from testosterone could affect breast cancer risk. In this study, called the Testosterone Implant Breast Cancer Prevention Study, the researchers wanted to see if using testosterone instead of the hormones in BHRT — estrogen and progesterone — to treat menopausal symptoms would increase the risk of breast cancer. Since March 2008, 1,268 postmenopausal women with no history of breast cancer who had menopausal symptoms were treated with a testosterone pellet implanted under the skin about every 3 months. None of the women were taking other forms of HRT. The women were about 52 years old when the first pellet was implanted.

Because doctors believe that estradiol converted from testosterone could affect breast cancer risk, some of the women were treated with pellets that also contained the aromatase inhibitor Arimidex (chemical name: anastrozole). Aromatase inhibitors are the most common type of hormonal therapy medicines used to lower the risk of breast cancer recurrence in postmenopausal women diagnosed with early-stage hormone-receptor-positive breast cancer. Aromatase inhibitors work by blocking aromatase. In women who had the testosterone-Arimidex pellet implanted under the skin, less testosterone was converted into estradiol. You can ask your doctor about these pellets as they are readily available - for Ladies only! This study seems to show that using the testosterone implant, with or without Arimidex, actually lowered the risk of breast cancer.

Still, the researchers pointed out that the study didn't have a control group of similar women who didn't get testosterone implants. We can't say for sure if using testosterone implants to treat menopausal symptoms reduces the risk of breast cancer. The researchers also found that none of the women who developed breast cancer while being treated with the testosterone implant had a cancer recurrence. I thought that alone was cool! The testosterone implant caused only mild side effects in some women, including an increase in facial hair, hair thinning, and a mild increase in acne; at the same time, about half of the women said their skin improved while being treated with the implants. I see skin improvement, in women, in my practice as well. Women who were treated with the testosterone-Arimidex implant had no side effects related to Arimidex.

While these results are promising, they are still early results. If you do your own research, make sure what you are researching is bio-identical testosterone and estrogen, not synthetic. Most of the research has been done with synthetic hormones, therefore you may see the increases in cancers with these compounds.

Now onto the **heart and the cardiovascular system for men and women**. Something near and dear to my heart! Testosterone pellets have been shown to lower cholesterol over time. Chris' actual labs are posted on the website showing his reduction in cholesterol over a one-year period. Let's take a closer look, as this is in my wheelhouse!

There are eight common types of heart disease present in men and women. These types of heart disease include high blood pressure, coronary artery disease, cardiac arrest, congestive heart failure, arrhythmia, peripheral artery disease, stroke, and congenital heart disease.

Most people do not associate high blood pressure with heart disease, but it is the most common form. It comes from the force of blood pumping through veins causing undue pressure on veins, creating a high-stress environment that accelerates aging of the veins. People older than 40 are most diagnosed with high blood pressure. Often high blood pressure has no symptoms, but severe high blood pressure can result in a stroke. Eating less salt and exercising regularly are ways that men and women may be able to lower their blood pressure without medical intervention. Stress management, quitting smoking, and diuretics may also be able to help lower blood pressure. At this point in time, we are evaluating taking Chris off his blood pressure medication, we are close.

One of the causes of heart disease may be a decline in estrogen after aging. Studies have shown that estrogen has a protective effect on the coronary system, and the loss of it can be difficult for the body to adjust to. Along with estrogen decreasing, cholesterol also tends to increase, making things more difficult for cardiac health. By supplementing missing estrogen with BHRT, you may be able to reduce the risk of heart disease as well as the severity of heart disease.

In 2015, a study hit the news showing that testosterone therapy increased cardiovascular risk. This flawed study used inadequate amounts and often the wrong form of testosterone, did not evaluate male subjects' estrogen levels, did not properly individualize the testosterone dose and failed to consider significantly different baseline testosterone levels. These flaws rendered this study's findings meaningless to aging men who properly optimize their testosterone and estrogen levels. In the paper published by JAMA (Journal of the American Medical Association), there was no report of the subjects' estradiol levels. If estradiol was not monitored during testosterone administration, this oversight means that the men receiving testosterone could have experienced a concurrent rise in estradiol levels. This may have compromised their cardiovascular health and could partially account for the increased risk observed in the testosterone-treated group.

Moving onto bones: Osteoporosis is the reduction of bone density and strength when the bone's mass decreases. The human body constantly takes in older bone tissue and renews it with fresh tissue. With osteoporosis, new bone creation does not occur frequently enough to match pace with old bone tissue reabsorption. The disorder affects men and women;

however, women are at a pointedly greater vulnerability than men of undergoing osteoporosis.

A primary function of estrogen in the body is ensuring that bones are protected. During aging, the quantity of estrogen in female bodies decreases. BHRT therapy provides a regular and constant supplementation of this vital hormone, reversing bone loss and renewing wellness to the core of your body.

Are you aware that osteoporosis can potentially be reduced and even reversed with BHRT? If you're on pellet therapy, data shows it builds strong bones, not hard bones that become brittle such as a side effect of the bisphosphonates, the name of the class of osteoporosis drugs. Also, the combination of vitamins A, D, and K with BHRT has been shown to increase bone mineral density by 8.3% a year. BHRT has helped numerous men and women relieve the symptoms of osteoporosis.

Onto the brain, not only does testosterone help your quality of sleep, but it also helps your mood. Testosterone also has a positive effect on amyloid plaque. What is amyloid plaque? It is laid down in your brain as a precursor to **dementia and**

Alzheimer's. If you're seventy or eighty and good health reading this, I would not walk; I would run to get your testosterone
pellets for this reason alone. There have been many veterans
with **PTSD** that BHRT has brought relief.

Let's talk about Alzheimer's for a minute: One of the causes for
the onset of Alzheimer's disease is thought to be an imbalance
of hormones. BHRT can put those hormones back in balance.
Your doctor can help you understand how BHRT can provide
symptom relief to you or a loved one. BHRT has been a crucial
component of Alzheimer's therapy for many men and women.

Alzheimer's disease is a disorder that is essentially a tissue
connective disorder in which the neural cells within the brain
degenerate and die, taking the memories they have built over
a lifetime with them. Alzheimer's therapy can be complicated,
but BHRT can make the process go as smoothly as possible.

In women, agitation and anger may present less readily than
in men with Alzheimer's. People with Alzheimer's disease may
repeat their own words, and the words of others, without
associated meaning. Confusion also may increase during the

evening hours. Eventually, as the disease progresses, the sufferer may be unable to form new memories or perform basic day-to-day adult living functions. BHRT can potentially relieve these symptoms. Though it is important to note that there are also potentially genetic and situational components that impact the likelihood and progression of Alzheimer's. Older people with little stimulation, such as those with a smaller social circle or less familial support, may have less resilience against the disease and may succumb more quickly to its progression, but BHRT may be able to help.

Let's go back to PTSD. Chris and I are big supporters of our veterans and a portion of this book's proceeds goes to support our heroes. Post-traumatic stress disorder (PTSD) in women may become more manageable with BHRT. BHRT therapy has helped numerous women with the symptoms of PTSD. Post-traumatic stress disorder, or PTSD, is a neurological condition brought on by witnessing or otherwise experiencing an emotionally and physically intense event. It is a very common condition, and more than three million Americans are diagnosed with it each year. The condition is treatable by a medical professional, although levels of success vary, and requires an accurate diagnosis. PTSD can last months or years, and treatment is typically restricted to psychotherapy and the use of prescribed medication to manage symptoms.

Post-traumatic stress disorder may cause nightmares, flash-backs and compulsive avoidance of situations that may remind the victim of the trauma. PTSD can have a crippling effect on the quality of life and impact every aspect of a person's life. For example, PTSD brought on from car wrecks can prevent sufferers from being able to ride in cars without significant dis-tress. Intense emotional reactions to everyday situations can be exhausting, leaving sufferers feeling depressed, isolated, and as if they may never be able to experience normalcy again. That's where BHRT therapy comes in. BHRT can help address hormonal imbalances caused by PTSD and return you to as normal a life as possible.

Let's take a minute and talk about men, **testosterone, and aro-matization**. This is basically breaking down testosterone and converting it into estrogen which is fine in good balance. This happens in a low percentage of men on BHRT. Your physician will help you with this, but a good rule of thumb will be the 5% rule. In round numbers, let's say your post pellet labs show a total testosterone level of 1,000 and your estradiol of 50, which would be a 5% ratio. That would be a good healthy number. Now let's say that ratio goes from 5% to 10%, same testosterone of 1,000 and now you have an estradiol of 100. This could be getting it into a concerning area that we would call aromatizing. Now, this is where it gets kind of tricky, and it's going to be on a physician to physician level on what to do. Every physician has a different thought process on aromatization. A good physician is going to ask you how you feel, you have three ranges of feelings. Range one is more in the semi rage, getting a little pissed off at somebody cutting you off in traffic and maybe getting testy with your wife. On the other side of that would be some feelings of sadness and mild depression and you might even get some erectile dysfunction. Then there's a place in the middle where you feel balanced with harmony and happiness in your life. If your estradiol is higher than 8% of your testosterone, or over say 70, more than likely your physician will want to knock that down with a drug called anastrozole, or an aromatase inhibitor. Make sure you're taking your dim twice a day, always! More on DIM in the nutraceutical section.

Chris and I have agreed not to mention anyone by name, quote, or leave links or references to articles and not to mention brand names or company names in the VPD book as to stay as informational and entertaining as possible. We have a website, YouTube, and Instagram as resources for all that. I do feel it is important for you to be armed with the truth about the safety of BHRT. Both estrogen and testosterone. Having the following data, both as a physician and patient, you will be armed with the truth.

The following are bullet points, a review and summation of testosterone from many published scientific articles on testosterone, prostate cancer, male sexual dysfunction, and male infertility.

- Testosterone is more than a male sex hormone
- Testosterone stimulates and maintains muscle and bone growth for example
- Low T puts men at increased risk for osteoporosis with advancing age
- Testosterone stimulates red blood cell production, helping to prevent anemia
- Testosterone levels are reduced in type 2 diabetes
- Therapy with testosterone can reduce LDL cholesterol, blood sugar, glycated hemoglobin, and insulin resistance.
- Men with low Testosterone die earlier than those with normal Testosterone

- Testosterone does not cause prostate cancer
- Prostate cancer cells behave less aggressively in the presence of testosterone
- Normal levels of testosterone may even turn out to be beneficial for men with prostate cancer
- Men with reductions in testosterone levels have an increased risk for prostate cancer

Estrogen

Before we get into estrogen, I just want to clarify a couple of things for you ladies out there. Guys we just had a nice talk about testosterone and aromatization, safety, etc. so it's their turn! Also, men read this as well - it will help you to be more sympathetic to your better half! As I mentioned before, peri and post-menopause can be quite debilitating. It can be a major interrupter in your day and night in the hot flashes and night sweats. When you wake up and your sweating at night for no apparent reason this is a result of testosterone deficiency thus the night sweats. The reason I point this out is that they are two separate physiological processes that are going on in your body. They are the result of two hormones being low so that's important to remember when you're thinking about how you're feeling and if you need testosterone or an estrogen pellet. Your physician will be more precise with you when you have this discussion so when you're talking to your physician about getting the hormone pellets, make sure that you clarify the fact that you have either night sweats or hot flashes or you could have both.

Now onto some misconceptions of estrogen. In the VDP, females only get pellets of testosterone, or estrogen, or both. While we are on the subject of estrogen, there are many misconceptions in the media and in physician's minds. You may have heard from your neighbor, your hairdresser, or your bartender, that estrogen causes cancer. Let me summarize why this has happened.

I want Chris to tell a story here as during the following time point, as now, I was practicing Cardiology and did not live this as Chris did. I will pick back up after Chris' story. Thank you, Dr. Pace! This is a true story! Approximately 15 years ago while I was a big pharma rep, I was a specialty rep with a concentration in women's health. It certainly made for interesting conversations on dates for sure! I was selling a synthetic combination hormone product for menopausal containing synthetic estrogen and progesterone. At the same time, a clinical trial was in full swing by the National Institutes of Health. This clinical trial was called the Women's Health Initiative. Let me just give you an overview of the study: They were trying to answer the question of the safety of hormone replacement in women. Keep in mind, this was done with synthetic, mostly horse urine derived hormones. I can't make this up! The Women's Health Initiative studied 27,347 U.S. women ages 50-79 who enrolled between 1993 and 1998. There were 16,608 women with an intact uterus in the trial of estrogen plus progestin and 10,739 without a uterus in the trial of estrogen-alone. Women with an intact uterus were enrolled in the estrogen plus progestin trial because of the need to add progestin to the therapy to protect against endometrial cancer. Of those who participated in the original trial, 81 percent agreed to continue follow-up after the planned end of the trials. The WHI compared the rates of developing coronary heart disease including a heart attack, stroke, breast cancer, blood clots in the lungs, colorectal cancer, endometrial cancer, hip fracture, and death among women who were assigned to hormones versus women who were assigned to placebo study pills. Again, keep in mind that they were using synthetic hormones and not bioidenticals and the women were taking them by mouth, and not inserted in adipose tissue. That could be a book looking at the metabolism of synthetic hormones by mouth and the side effects.

In the estrogen and progesterone arm, they saw slight increases in the above-mentioned including cancer so, they decided to reveal that information to the press. So out of the blue, the nightly news announced that hormones cause cancer! As you can imagine, every woman on hormones was calling their OBGYN office, the next morning - scared to death - rightfully so! Every OBGYN office was calling my flip phone cell phone, - rightfully so as well. It sent these OBGYN offices into a tailspin as they could not handle all the calls. The reaction of physicians and patients was just to stop all postmenopausal HRT altogether. You can imagine the hysteria!

Then a retrospective look at the data a few years later showed the details of the trial showed one arm using progesterone called Medroxyprogesterone acetate. This (MPA) was the culprit! It was identified years later, that didn't hit the news or the media or the physician's office. Therefore, many women have suffered without hormones. Due to this information circulating out there, that is why you may hear that hormones cause cancer. This is an important story for you ladies out there as you need to be armed with the truth! OK - Back to Dr. Pace as he further discusses estrogen.

So now that we have that cleared up, let's talk about other forms of estrogen in the marketplace. There is systemic estrogen — which comes in a pill, skin patch, gel, cream, or spray form — they can be effective for treatment and relief of troublesome menopausal symptoms like hot flashes. Estrogen can also ease vaginal symptoms, such as dryness, itching, burning, and discomfort with intercourse. Keep in mind these products do not give you steady blood levels like BHRT. Some data also suggest that estrogen can decrease the risk of heart disease when taken early in the postmenopausal years. Systemic estrogen helps protect against the bone-thinning disease called osteoporosis. However, doctors usually recommend medications called bisphosphonates to treat osteoporosis. If you look at the data with BHRT and Vitamin D - more on this later, patients will experience an increase of bone mineral density of 8.3% a year on this therapy. Keep in mind this with a combination of testosterone. There are also low-dose vaginal products. Low-dose vaginal preparations of estrogen — which come in cream, tablet or ring form — can effectively treat vaginal symptoms and some urinary symptoms while minimizing absorption into the body. Low-dose vaginal preparations do not help with hot flashes, night sweats or protection against osteoporosis.

THIS IS IMPORTANT LADIES!! If you haven't had your uterus removed, your doctor will typically prescribe estrogen along with progesterone or progestin (progesterone-like medication). This is because estrogen alone, when not balanced by progesterone, can stimulate the growth of the lining of the uterus, *increasing the risk of uterine cancer.* If you have had your uterus removed (hysterectomy), you don't need to take progesterone. Literally, hundreds of clinical studies have provided evidence that systemic hormone therapy (estrogen with or without progestogen) effectively helps such conditions as hot flashes, vaginal dryness, night sweats, and bone loss. These benefits can lead to improved sleep, sexual relations, and quality of life. So hopefully after reading this, you will realize that bioidentical estrogen pellets are the way to go. Ask your doctor what is right for you and I hope this is laid to rest any fears you may have in this area. Let's move on to another big one!

Thyroid

This is a big one! Again, many great books are written on thyroid and iodine alone. This is the section of the book where endocrinologists will want to throw stones at me as this goes against the grain of their thinking and against the grain of big pharma. I am about the truth, so here goes!

Let's look at some parameters of the thyroid so you get an understanding of the whole picture - the blood tests for thyroid function—TSH, total T4, free T3—are an important part of diagnosing and treating thyroid disorders. While some conclusions can be drawn from a single test, a combination of test results is usually needed to establish the full nature of your thyroid health. By comparing the values of thyroid tests, a doctor can determine whether a person has hypothyroidism (low thyroid function) or hyperthyroidism (overactive thyroid). Figuring out what the various names and numbers mean can be complicated but taking the time to learn them can help you better manage your disease along with your doctor, if disease is present.

The purpose of thyroid testing is to measure the so-called "markers" of thyroid health. These are substances not only produced by the thyroid gland but other organs that regulate thyroid function. For example, the pituitary gland produces a hormone known as thyroid-stimulating hormone (TSH), which regulates how much of the hormones triiodothyronine (T3) and thyroxine (T4) are produced by the thyroid gland. The interrelationship of these and other values can tell you a lot about how well or how poorly your thyroid gland is functioning.

I can't tell you how many women and men that I talk to say they feel awful. They've gone to their doctor and their thyroid is "normal". In your labs, you have two main areas of the thyroid. I'll try to keep this simple for you: you have T4 and T3. T4 is in your thyroid and it can be treated with a product called Synthroid. Certainly, you've heard of this drug, as it is the highest-grossing pharmaceutical product ever and it does affect how people feel. However, T4 is only 25% bioavailable. What does this mean? In simple terms, this algorithm is only 25% effective, or you may feel 25% better. What you need to look at, and your doctor knows this on the VDP is T3 levels. Now keep in mind if you go back to your endocrinologist and start talking about T3 they're going to laugh at you be-e big pharma has them convinced them that T4 is the way to go. Just giving you a head up here: Get your T3 level checked, and you want it over four as the lab value. This can be treated very easily with an affordable prescription and it's only under $30 a month at the pharmacy. This will be on the website as I am keeping this book purely for entertainment and education and no branded products or companies will be mentioned here. The take-home message here is real simple - get your T3 looked at and have this discussion with your physician - cool?

We will cover iodine briefly in the nutraceutical section. Let's have a discussion here as this is critical to Thyroid support. Iodine is an element that is needed to produce thyroid hormone. The body does not make iodine, so it is an essential part of your diet. Iodine is found in various foods. Iodine is present naturally in soil and seawater. The availability of iodine in foods differs in various regions of the world. Individuals in the United States can maintain adequate iodine in their diet by using iodized table salt, by eating foods high in iodine, particularly dairy products, seafood, meat, breads, eggs, and by taking a multivitamin containing iodine. I have Chris taking an iodine supplement because he uses Himalayan pink salt and is vegan. Also, the amount of iodine in foods is not listed on food packaging in the U.S., and it can be difficult to identify sources of iodine in foods.

If you do not have enough iodine in your body, you cannot make enough thyroid hormone. Thus, iodine deficiency can lead to enlargement of the thyroid or goiter, hypothyroidism, and intellectual disabilities in infants and children whose mothers were iodine deficient during pregnancy. Before the 1920s, iodine deficiency was common in the Great Lakes, Appalachian, and Northwestern U.S. regions and in most of Canada. Prevention of iodine deficiency by the introduction of iodized salt has virtually eliminated iodine deficiency and the so-called "goiter belt" in these areas. However, many other parts of the world do not have enough iodine available through their diet and iodine deficiency continues to be an important public health problem globally. Approximately 30% of the world's population remains at risk for iodine deficiency.

Iodine deficiency is diagnosed across populations and not specifically in individuals. In the United States, iodine status has remained generally adequate in since the 1940s although studies have shown that urinary iodine levels dropped by about half between the early 1970s and the early 1990s, and most recently mild iodine deficiency has re-emerged in pregnant women. Iodine deficiency remains a major issue in other parts of the world, including parts of Europe, Africa, and Asia. The take-home message here is we are not getting enough from our diet. Speak to your doctor about iodine supplementation and make sure you are getting a pure source from a reputable supplier.

Progesterone

OK, Men - I'll give you a pass here - go grab a beer - wait - have you started the protocol yet? OK then grab a martini and read the testosterone section again as the following is pretty much for the wonderful ladies out there. Ladies - MUST READ!! Before we dive into progesterone I just wanted to make sure that you get the important take-home message upfront here - here if *you have a uterus and you are on estrogen therapy you must take your progesterone, this is not negotiable.* Why? You take progesterone in order to prevent endometrial cancer. That should be enough said in this chapter but let's discuss it for a second.

Let's look and see how progesterone works in the body. This is a stretch from Cardiology, but an important part of the VDP for the ladies! Progesterone is one of the steroid hormones. It is secreted by the corpus luteum, an endocrine gland. The female body produces this after ovulation and during the second half of the menstrual cycle. Progesterone prepares the endometrium for the potential of pregnancy after ovulation. It triggers the lining to thicken to accept a fertilized egg. It also prohibits the muscle contractions in the uterus that would cause the body to reject an egg. While the body is producing high levels of progesterone, the body will not ovulate. If the woman does not become pregnant, the corpus luteum breaks down, lowering the progesterone levels in the body. This change sparks menstruation. If the body does conceive, progesterone continues to stimulate the body to provide the blood vessels in the endometrium that will feed the growing fetus. The hormone also prepares the limit of the uterus further so it can accept the fertilized egg. Once the placenta develops, it also begins to secrete progesterone, supporting the corpus luteum. This causes the levels to remain elevated throughout the pregnancy, so the body does not produce more eggs. It also helps prepare the breasts for milk production.

To boil this down, ladies, you need progesterone. A simple way to think about this - in the words of one of my hormone mentors - estrogen in the uterus is the fertilizer and progesterone is the lawnmower. They need to be in balance with each other. Your VDP physician will know all this and it is an important discussion to have.

Talk to your doctor about synthetic "progestin" and compounded progesterone! Controlled studies and most observational studies published in the last five years suggest that the addition of progestins (synthetic progesterone) to hormone replacement therapy, particularly in a continuous combined regimen, increases the risk of breast cancer compared to estrogen alone. While the results of clinical trials may accurately assess the risks associated with synthetic progestin compounds and estrogen/progestin combinations, the data does not reflect what might have been the result had natural progesterone been used instead of synthetic progesterone. We discussed this a bit when Chris mentioned the WHI study. When discussing progesterone, it is important to understand the difference between natural progesterone and synthetic progesterone analogs called progestins. Progestogens are an umbrella term for both natural progesterone and synthetic progestins because they all have progestational effects in the uterus. Just ask your doctor about compounded micronized progesterone.

Natural progesterone is synthesized in the laboratory from either soybeans or the Mexican wild yam (Dioscorea villosa). The process was discovered in the 1930s by Pennsylvania State University professor Russell Marker, who transformed diosgenin from wild yams into natural progesterone. Natural progesterone refers to bioidentical hormone products that have a molecular structure identical to the hormones our bodies manufacture naturally. Just as the estradiol pellets and testosterone pellets are bioidentical as well. The process of micronization allows for steady and even absorption of the medication. Micronized progesterone is available only through a doctor's prescription. An alternative is natural progesterone creams sold over the counter worldwide. Just be careful here and listen to your doctor as progesterone is a large molecule and the cream could have questionable absorption and therefore questionable uterine protection. Both the micronized progesterone and commercially available progesterone creams contain bioidentical progesterone. Again, listen to your doctor.

To summarize progesterone, it has many functions in the body include:

- maintaining the uterine lining and preventing excess tissue buildup
- inhibiting breast tissue overgrowth
- increasing metabolism and promoting weight loss
- balancing blood sugar levels
- acting as a natural diuretic
- normalizing blood clotting
- stimulating the production of new bone
- enhancing the action of thyroid hormones
- alleviating depression and reducing anxiety
- promoting normal sleep patterns
- preventing cyclical migraines
- restoring proper cell oxygen levels
- improving libido.5-16 (Bonus ladies!)

The take-home message is to speak to your doctor about the need for progesterone, the correct form and correct dose for you.

Peptides

3

The following is very exciting stuff. I, Dr. Pace, am currently exploring a peptide regimen that will work for
me. Peptides have so many uses in medicine, and
there are currently over 7000 compounds out there. Why have
you not heard of them? Either they are generic forms of drugs,
or they are natural and cannot be patented. Remember to follow the money in medicine! For this section, I have asked Chris
to do the heavy lifting as he has lived this as a patient and give
you his personal experience along with some research that has
been done in this area. So please take it away Chris!

Wow! Thank you, Dr. Pace! What an honor! I can't decide if
this is my favorite chapter of this book or is it hormones? You

decide and please let me know. Being that I am currently on peptides and BHRT and the fact that I feel doubly amazing on the two has me throwing them into a tie. Think of them as peanut butter and jelly, or peas and carrots! They just go so well together. Maybe it's that my prediction that peptides, again my opinion, will revolutionize the landscape of medicine - along with BHRT. Just wait until your hormones are optimized, you are on say a combination of sermorelin and GHRP 2 and you go to the gym - only then will you understand how you feel! Yes, ladies too! Like many chapters in this book, someone could write a book on peptides! For the sake of time and your value in this book, we will discuss a handful of peptides instead of 7000 and we will keep the conversation around changing your body from fat to muscle. Sound good?

Let's dive in! I'm so excited!! Your life, as mine has, is about to change!! Peptides are short-chain amino acids that are building blocks for proteins. They can also be signaling molecules for other processes in your body. Let's look at the main function here: the endogenous (from within) production of human growth hormone. Let's stop and talk about human growth hormone (HGH) for a second. HGH, also called somatotropin, is secreted by the anterior lobe of the pituitary gland. It stimulates the growth of essentially all tissues of the body, including bone. HGH is synthesized and secreted by anterior pituitary cells called somatotrophs, which release between one and two milligrams of the hormone each day, then decrease as we age. HGH is vital for normal physical growth in children; its levels rise progressively during childhood and peak during the growth spurt that occurs in puberty. You may have heard of HGH injections in the bodybuilding community or the anti-aging world. HGH injections are loaded with controversy, available on the black market, and highly scrutinized by the FDA. When the bodybuilding community found out about this it was all the rage for a while. Then the FDA came down on the entire industry and now it is highly regulated. Physicians are leery to prescribe HGH it and it can be prohibitively expensive. I just wanted to cover this, so you know the difference between the HGH that your body produces naturally and HGH injections.

Now let's look at some of the technical aspects of peptides: First the definition - Peptides, from the Greek language, peptós "digested"; derived from péssein "to digest" are short chains of amino acid monomers linked by peptide (amide) bonds. The covalent chemical bonds are formed when the carboxyl group of one amino acid reacts with the amino group of another. Sorry about all that - who knows - there could be a scientist reading this book! Oh - peptides are also present in your skin and are the building blocks of healthy skin. Collagen is a protein comprised of long segments of amino acids arranged like a chain. When collagen breaks down, short segments of amino acids are formed. These are the tiny proteins and active molecules known as peptides. Peptides in skincare can provide significant anti-aging benefits. Ladies - ask your doctor about these forms of peptides. When you use this form of peptides with estrogen pellets the results can be amazing in women for skincare - men too, but we really are not into skincare for the most part.

Peptides are smaller than proteins. Traditionally, peptides are defined as molecules that consist of between 2 and 50 amino acids, whereas proteins are made up of 50 or more amino acids.

So currently Sermorelin seems to be the most common peptide used in clinics. Very popular now are the combination of two or three peptides in one injection. We'll start with Sermorelin with ghrp 2 and ghrp-6. At the time of this writing, there

has been some buzz around the availability of this combination, and quite honestly you may not want to start here, and
I will tell you why - again keeping this book open, honest, and
real. Let's break this down and start with a discussion around
Sermorelin. While this is a phenomenal peptide, there may be
better options depending on the price point and the advice of
your physician. Then again there are many reasons why this
could be a great place for you to start your peptide journey.

First, let's get the technical stuff out of the way for Sermorelin.
This is good information if you have a technical side to you
so here goes. Sermorelin acetate (sermorelin) is the acetate
salt of an amidated synthetic 29- amino acid peptide (GRF
1-29 NH 2) that corresponds to the amino-terminal segment
of the naturally occurring human growth hormone-releasing
hormone (GHRH or GRF) consisting of 44 amino acid residues.
Sermorelin is the structurally truncated analog of Growth Hormone Releasing Hormone (GHRH). That's why I put the HGH
section above, so this could make more sense and you can see
how this ties together. Sermorelin consists of the first 29 amino acids of the naturally occurring neurohormone that is produced in the hypothalamus. Also, note that Sermorelin is the
most widely used member of the GHRH analog drug class. It

can significantly promote the synthesis and release of growth hormone (GH) from cells in the pituitary gland, improving the serum concentrations of GH and subsequently insulin-like growth factor 1 (IGF-1) in animals and humans. By the way - make sure your doctor checks your IGF-1 level before starting peptide therapy - your doctor can discuss this with you.

Remember how Dr. Pace said hormones are like the conductor in a symphony? Sermorelin can influence the concert of hormonal signals that affect GH secretion from the anterior pituitary including GHRH, somatostatin, and insulin-like growth factor (IGF) and others. Let me take a moment and give the scientific explanation of what happens in the body. You don't have to grasp all this, but your doctor may be new to this so here goes.

The positive and negative opposing regulation of growth hormone by GHRH and somatostatin, respectively, creates a rhythmic-circadian pattern of HGH secretion. Thus, modification of both pulse amplitude and frequency of HGH secretion results from Sermorelin administration. After sermorelin stimulates the release of HGH from the pituitary gland, it increases the synthesis of IGF-1 in the liver and peripheral tissues.

Sermorelin acts on the growth hormone-releasing hormone receptor (GHRHr) in the pituitary to regulate cellular activities. GHRHr is the natural receptor for the endogenous hormone, GHRH, and for sermorelin. This receptor regulates growth hormone release directly by stimulation and indirectly by feedback relationships with somatostatin. Got all that? Almost done with the technical stuff - I just find this fascinating! Sermorelin is readily degraded after reaching the bloodstream, having a biological half-life of approximately 10-20 min. Therefore, administered at bedtime. Three (3) mcg/kg subcutaneous injections of Sermorelin have been reported to simulate a naturally occurring GHRH mediated GH release responses.

Your doctor will discuss mixing and dosing in detail with you. In short, it is just a diabetic (small) needle that you really don't feel - honestly! At this point in my journey, I have had around 180 injections, and all is good, this also includes the HCG injections as well!

This is really cool! In addition to increasing production and secretion, GHRH also affects sleep patterns by increasing the amount of slow-wave sleep (SWS) while augmenting sleep-related GH secretion and reducing cortisol secretion. I sleep like a baby - REM every night!!

The doctors that are new to this will want to know the Mechanism of Action or MOA: Sermorelin essentially mimics the hypothalamic peptide, GHRH. Sermorelin acts directly on the pituitary stimulating the somatotroph cell's ability to produce and secrete GH. Sermorelin increases the proliferation of somatotroph cells during development. With the increase of serum GH, downstream effects occur. A notable hormone that is commonly used as a surrogate for growth hormone therapy, insulin-like growth factor 1 (IGF-1), is known to increase with the administration of Sermorelin. IGF-I negatively regulates GHRH-mediated GH secretion. Sermorelin can influence the concert of hormonal signaling that affects the GH axis. GH secretion from the anterior pituitary is regulated by GHRH, somatostatin, and GH secretagogues.

What does this all mean? Sermorelin tells your pituitary gland to produce HGH in your body to help you lose fat and gain muscle while following the vodka diet protocol (VDP). I know that was a mouthful! I am just trying to entertain doctors, PAs, ARNPs, teachers, firemen, and bartenders, etc. We will need to take those technical breaks every now and then, but I think it does give you a good technical synopsis and some layman's terms of how all this works and comes together in the VDP.

Now let's go on to the combination that I took for a month. After I tell you about the other two components, I will tell you my story. I'm doing all this to help you to go down the right pathway so that you won't make the same mistakes I have. I also want you to get the results I have achieved. Now let's do a little shallow dive into GHRP-2 and GHRP-6 or Growth Hormone Releasing Peptide. GHRP-2 has been widely studied for its helpfulness and action as a growth hormone secretagogue (GHS), meaning it stimulates the secretion of growth hormone. This is a hexapeptide with potent properties. It is known to promote hunger and appetite by stimulating Ghrelin release. This will also lead us into a discussion concerning ghrelin, the hunger hormone. Ghrelin has been shown to have two major effects, stimulating both GH secretion and appetite/meal initiation. Sort of like a double-edged sword! GHRP-2 has been extensively studied for its utility as a growth hormone secretagogue (GHS). ... However, whether GHRP-2 can also stimulate appetite in humans when administered acutely is not known. That's what the scientists say - I say a big Texas "hell yes!" It stimulates hunger like cardboard hunger - Like if you are in between me and the refrigerator your arm goes next hungry! Just keep in mind I am basing this hunger on the combination of sermorelin, ghrp-6, and ghrp-2. At the time of writing this, there have been some rumblings of this combination being not so popular with the FDA. We wanted to include it here to be transparent and real. By the time you read this, they may or may not be available. Please check the website for an update on this. Spoiler alert - In my opinion, GHRP - 6 is the hunger culprit here! Let's move into ghrp-6.

GHRP 6

I will call this the hunger peptide! Some technical stuff, then more on my story: Growth hormone-releasing peptide 6 (GHRP-6) (developmental code name SKF-110679), also known as growth hormone-releasing hexapeptide, is one of several synthetic met-enkephalin analogs that include unnatural D-amino acids, were developed for their growth hormone-releasing activity and are called growth hormone secretagogues. They lack opioid activity but are potent stimulators of growth hormone (GH) release. These secretagogues are distinct from growth hormone-releasing hormone (GHRH) in that they share no sequence relation and derive their function through activation of a completely different receptor. This receptor was originally called the growth hormone secretagogue receptor (GHSR), but due to subsequent discoveries, the hormone ghrelin is now considered the receptor's natural endogenous ligand, and it has been renamed as the ghrelin receptor. Therefore, these GHSR agonists act as synthetic ghrelin mimetics. Therefore, the hunger peptide! Sorry, it took all that to explain this but this is important so you realize why a barn will taste good if you get on the GHRP. If you are a bodybuilder or chronically underweight, I could see a good utility here.

It has been discovered that when GHRP-6 and insulin are administered simultaneously, GH response to GHRP-6 is increased. However, the consumption of carbohydrates and/or dietary fats, around the administration window of GH secretagogues significantly blunts the GH release. A recent study in normal mice showed significant differences in body composition, muscle growth, glucose metabolism, memory, and cardiac function in the mice being administered the GHRP-6 (2). There are still many questions regarding this new compound. I put this here because your clinic may advise against eating carbs at night and using GHRPs. Now you know why. I believe it should be standard fair not to eat or drink carbs after a certain hour, but even more, a reason to do so here.

I do my peptide injections right after brushing my teeth last thing before bed, so talk to your doctor and see what works well for you. I think most will agree with this, as GH is secreted at night. Also, a possible side effect of these peptides is better to sleep. Also, BHRT gives me an amazing sleep pattern throughout this entire process. Hopefully, your sleep will greatly improve, having a profound impact on your quality of life and your health.

A little more of my story on Sermorelin, GHRP 2 and 6. Four words sum this up hunger, hunger, hunger, and gains. Hunger - cardboard hunger! Enough said about that - you get the point. Muscle gains - well maybe not actual tissue in one month, but an increase in strength, reps, etc. in the gym, which is way cool for the purpose of the VDP. There was no doubt about it, I could look in the mirror and see little muscles popping out that I never knew were there, my veins were bigger too. I don't want to sound too down on this combo. Maybe you are not a food addict like me and can control the hunger aspect here. Maybe you are underweight and just looking to gain muscle. Maybe you are into bulking and cutting, and maybe a little more advanced - then this would be a great combo for you.

More than likely your clinic will have you on peptides for 3-month cycles. I did this combo for one month and then took a one-week break and moved on the next combo. Also, there are two schools of thought - take your peptides straight through for 3 months then cycle off. Again, listen to your doctor - many will recommend weekends off or 2 days with no peptides. This worked for me - I try to take off one or two days from the gym so no gym - no injection the night before - cool? Also, I am looking out for your wallet here and this practice will extend your "peptide time." Again, listen to your doctor, PA, ARNP!! Some experts say to do peptides for 90 days straight and some say take weekends off, so listen to your doctor. This what I call 90/5/2. 90/5/2 is a script for 90 days of therapy, 5 days on the therapy followed by 2 days off. This clearly will last more than 90 days, therefore, it's a nice little trick to stretch your wallet. Any trick to stretch your wallet I will share as you, the patient is the most important element in all of this!

Sermorelin, GHRP-2 and L-Theanine

Before we start, in certain places in this book, I would like to give credit where credit is due. This combination was introduced to me by a dear person, we'll just call her CK for now. CK is a brilliant PA and has been an instrumental part of my life while writing this book. Dr. Pace and I just want to give her credit here and thank her for a brilliant idea of this combination. This combination works great and my hunger here has been elevated, yet controllable. So, therefore it is only my opinion that ghrp-6 has a greater effect on ghrelin then ghrp-2, therefore, less effect on hunger. Now keep in mind ghrp-2 does increase your hunger but trust me, it is much more manageable.

With the addition of L-theanine, this combination really helps you sleep as well. Of course, this sleep is all amplified being on the hormone pellets. You will hear me and Dr. Pace, throughout this book mention quality, deep REM sleep is the cornerstone of your health and the VDP. Also, go light on the vodka as too much is never good for sleep!

I believe we have discussed sermorelin and ghrp-2 previously. Let's take a look at l-theanine. First, let's do our famous little shallow clinical dive here, and then I can tell you more about how this combination has helped me. First, L-theanine is not a peptide, but an amino acid. L-theanine promotes relaxation and facilitates sleep by contributing to a few changes in the brain and boosts levels of GABA and other calming brain chemicals. L-theanine elevates levels of GABA, as well as serotonin and dopamine. These chemicals are known as neurotransmitters, and they work in the brain to regulate emotions, mood, concentration, alertness, and sleep, as well as appetite, energy, and cognitive skills. Increasing levels of these calming brain chemicals promote relaxation and can help with sleep. You can see why this would be a great combination! At the same time, it is increasing chemicals that promote feelings of calm, L-theanine also reduces levels of chemicals in the brain that are linked to stress and anxiety. This may also be a way that L-theanine can protect brain cells against stress and age-related damage. It also enhances alpha brain waves. Alpha brain waves are associated with a state of "wakeful relaxation." That's the state of mind you experience when meditating, being creative, or letting your mind wander in daydreaming. More on meditating in the sauna later. Alpha waves are also present during <u>REM</u> sleep. L-theanine appears to trigger the release of <u>alpha-waves</u>, which enhances relaxation, focus, and <u>creativity</u>.

I have done this combination for 3 months. I just cannot say enough about it. After all, hopefully, my pictures tell the story. Again, the VDP is about a personalized evidence-based proto-col that you and your clinic need to put together to see what works best for you. Just because this was the most successful combination for me does not mean it would be the best for you. This is not a one-size-fits-all protocol. You find out what works best for your body. We also take into account the finan-cial aspect of all this. I'm not rich and chances are you aren't either. Yes, most of this costs money so finances will come into consideration based on what you are prescribed and what you can afford. I will do a deeper dive into how much this all costs later in the book, in The Plan chapter.

Ipamorelin/Sermorelin/ Theanine Sub-Lingual

OK, all you needle-phobics! I have the answer for you! Yes, you can take peptides without a needle! The other day a buddy, Tom was visiting my house and I have a section of my kitchen that resembles more of a pharmacy than a kitchen, complete with vials and needles. He inquired as to what was going on there and I began to describe the VDP. He just held up his hand and said he was out on anything that involves needles. I understand, so we have a solution for you! I just put this little tablet under my tongue at bedtime and let it dissolve. Talk to your doctor about this method of delivery as some are not in agreement with this. Also, you need about 50 times the active ingredient as it is not being injected into your body. Either way, it's nice to have an alternative here and like everything this book, I wanted to try it. Just due to the timing of the release of the book, I just did this for about 3 weeks. I can report all positive here - great sleep, strength in the gym, etc.

Since you are familiar with sermorelin and theanine, let's discuss ipamorelin. Ipamorelin is Growth Hormone Releasing

Peptide (GHRP). Like GHRP 2 and GHRP 6. Think of ipamorelin as a cousin to sermorelin, as they have similar traits and characteristics. Just like Sermorelin, Ipamorelin is a secretagogue. Ipamorelin causes some response by binding the cellular receptors. I mention cellular receptors as these are the receptors that you want to give a break to while on the VDP. Now back to the point - ipamorelin stimulates the pituitary gland to produce the growth hormone into the bloodstream, sound familiar? In most cases, ipamorelin works in the liver and the brain, and this makes it suitable for anti-aging effects. Again, not a big fan of the word anti-aging but I think you get the point. Compared to other peptides, ipamorelin is the mildest GHRP, therefore great in combination therapy. Since it targets a specific growth hormone pulse and heightens ghrelin, ipamorelin is like GHRP-6. Nevertheless, unlike the GHRP-6, ipamorelin doesn't stimulate hunger anything close to GHRP 6. Therefore, I wanted to try this one and compare it. Since it is a versatile hormone, ipamorelin is more suitable as a bedtime dose as all mentioned here are prescribed at bedtime. This is cool - despite being the mildest GHRP, ipamorelin is not the weakest. It is the longest lasting GHRP, and it is more potent at higher doses. Ipamorelin also functions as a slow-building hormone just like the natural growth hormone. This makes it the healthiest peptide in some people's opinion.

MK-677 or Ibutamoren

In all fairness and transparency, I have not tried this peptide at the time of writing this. It is most definitely the next peptide I will try, and will keep in touch on Instagram and YouTube on this one.

Ibutamoren, formerly known as Nutrobal or MK-677, is a newer player in the world of peptides. Its benefits have not been officially confirmed yet, but more than a few people swear by it and I am aware of a few clinics that are prescribing it. Even though it's mainly associated with bodybuilders, people with disabilities and hormone deficiencies benefit from it as well. Many people often mistake Ibutamoren for a steroid, which it is not. It is not a typical growth stimulator either. Ibutamoren is a secretagogue that mimics ghrelin, a growth stimulator. Remember this discussion from GHRP 6? It increases levels of the growth hormone in the plasma. However, it does not affect cortisol levels, which is great. Drugs that increase cortisol levels are usually very effective and fast, but they usually have terrible side-effects. This Peptide is not like that, its effects are positive and most long-lasting.

Originally named Nutrobal, Ibutamoren first started as a hormone booster that was used to help people with insulin and growth hormone deficiencies. The first brand that started producing it is Oratrope. Back then, its status was 'experimental'. It quickly gained popularity because of bodybuilders who started using it to gain mass. Although the VDP is not a bodybuilding protocol, I have to hand it to the bodybuilding community as they have been pioneers in the Peptide arena. Basically, Ibutamoren enabled them to quickly gain muscle and get rid of fat. It's no wonder that it blew up so quickly. No wonder why I want to try it! It sounds like a neat concept for an old guy like me or the peri-post menopausal women needing an edge.

Like Dr. Pace and I have said, this book is not about a bunch of scientific reference articles, but more of a true story. With that being said, Ibutamoren has been shown to improve lean body mass in a study. In the Rochester University study, a group of overall healthy 60-year-olds took Ibutamoren supplements for three months. I like the fact that they used 60-year-olds and not 30-year-olds! Most of them had shown a significant increase in lean body mass.

Another study, in Seoul, they tested the properties of Ibutamoren. This time, the subjects were women aged 22–46 years old, and this time, they were following a diet prescribed by the researchers. These subjects also showed major improvement in lean body mass. In addition, they also experienced a major fat loss. This leads to a point in the VDP. The VDP protocol does not need to be reserved for the say the over 40 crowd. These peptides are a great idea if your testosterone and hormone levels are where they should be and you are, say, under 40. This study shows good success in this age group without the need for BHRT. If your friend needs an edge on the scale or in the gym and they are younger than you, give them this book!

This VDP is not designed for teens or the college crowd, Ibutamoren was also proven to successfully treat growth hormone deficiency in both adults and children. One Chilean study treated 18 prepubescent children who suffered from this deficiency with Ibutamoren. The results were surprisingly positive — they were able to make up for the deficiency. And not just that, it was able to do so without affecting the cortisol, insulin, thyroxine, thyrotropin, or prolactin levels.

Remember our discussion on bone health and testosterone and Vitamin D? That was a few martini's ago, but when it comes to bone mineral density BMD, Ibutamoren has also shown success. There are more than a few studies on this topic. One tested obese men while others tested menopausal women and elders. All of them proved that Ibutamoren accelerates bone turnover and increases bone density. BMD improvement shows up in about a year. This is just way cool for the bones!

Although the VDP is not an anti-aging program, and you really cannot stop aging, it seems to be a buzz word that sounds like a cool concept. With that being said, Ibutamoren has anti-aging like properties and slows down muscle wasting. An interesting study in Israel backs this up. Any Orthopedic doctors out there? The researchers included elderly patients with hip fractures. After a few months, the subjects that took Ibutamoren daily were more successful at stair climbing and had fewer falls than those who took the placebo. They quickly regained their speed of motion. Basically, Ibutamoren can help patients recover faster from their injuries and get their strength back. We have covered pediatrics to the elderly here!

During most phases of the VDP, sleep and cognitive function can also improve, also true with Ibutamoren. Not only has it been shown to prevent cognitive decline that comes naturally with old age but also can enhance memory capacity. I cannot wait to try this peptide! Remember the discussion on HGH production by the pituitary and peptides? Ibutamoren also prolongs the REM stage of sleep which is way cool!

Oddly enough, Ibutamoren can also help regenerate tissue faster. One Texas study tested Ibutamoren on children who had severe burn injuries. The patients who took Ibutamoren took much less time to heal than those who didn't. Scientists say that the reason behind this is the Ibutamoren's effect on the growth hormone.

So that will wrap up Ibutamoren/MK-677. Are you seeing a common theme so far with these peptides and hormones? Fascinating science and again I cannot wait to try this one. As I said I will share results on Instagram and YouTube and please, I hope you will share with Dr. Pace and myself your results with all phases of the VDP. We want to create a like-minded community of positive people making positive changes in their lives.

CJC 1295

In closing, CJC 1295 is worthy of mentioning for sure. At the time of writing this, I have not tried this peptide as it is in my queue. Like we mentioned before, stay tuned to us online and I will share these results as well. For now, let's discuss this peptide as you may see it as DAC:GRF also in some circles.

CJC 1295 is a synthetically produced peptide that can increase your plasma growth hormone levels. Like most of the peptides, we have mentioned, CJC 1295 is usually injected into your body via a subcutaneous injection. In the VDP, your belly button will feel like a pincushion! As I said, CJC 1295 is also sometimes referred to as DAC:GRF or growth hormone-releasing factor. DAC or Drug Affinity Complex is added to this peptide in order to increase the half-life of CJC-1295. We could have a long discussion about DAC, the simple explanation is that DAC binds to proteins to prevent them from breaking down quickly. So that is one reason why I want to try this one, and here is a reason why maybe not. CJC 1295 can increase your IGF-1 levels and GH (growth hormone) levels. Remember our discussion on IGF-1? Again, I am not too concerned about this due to my diet. As I mentioned, Dr. Pace and I will keep you up to date from the experts on IGF-1 levels and peptides.

Initially, CJC 1295 was developed to treat diseases and medical conditions for patients who had muscle disorders, diseases, and burn victims. CJC 1295 has drawn many individuals like athletes from around the globe for its incredible benefits and minimal side effects to enhance their performance on the field and in the gym. These are just a few of the benefits which CJC-1295 will deliver upon. It is a long-acting GHRH analog (growth hormone-releasing hormone). I like this aspect, as a rule, most peptides are very short-acting. Therapeutic effects are increased because of this, and users require fewer injections in comparison to other growth hormones. These are just a few of the benefits CJC-1295 users will appreciate in comparison to other growth hormone injections available on the market. As always, follow your doctor's advice on the dosing and administration of this peptide.

More good news - when it comes to CJC-1295 with DAC, the main CJC-1295 effects are present as the growth hormone relates to the stimulation of the pituitary gland. (Peptides 101) An increase in vasodilation is often associated with the surge of the growth hormone into the user's body. This typically lasts for a period of 30 minutes to 2 hours, post-injection. Wait, did I say vasodilation? You may see this as a common theme in the VDP. Remember testosterone? This pretty much sums up why peptides and BHRT go so well together! Remember my story of how I feel in the gym while on peptides and BHRT? Well here is the answer - vasodilation - it's like icing on the cake - or like the olive in the martini!

OK, a few more points on CJC-1295. HGH levels also increase at the cellular level once CJC-1295 is injected. Research suggests this can lead to increased muscle strength, fat metabolism, and muscular mass. Ladies, improved skin-tone and muscle definition are also noted. In case we have not mentioned this, nothing in the VDP will make women bulk up. You really need levels of hormones and peptides that are way beyond this discussion.

Remember the combinations above that I mentioned? Growth hormone replacement peptides like GHRP 2 or 6 is typically used for synergistic effects, in conjunction with CJC-1295. This causes less of a cortisol surge, and prolactin, in comparison to GHRP 2. Like I mentioned, we are not getting into dosing here as that is a conversation with your doctor. One more note on CJC-1295, users report improved sleep. Like vasodilation, sleep is a common theme in the VDP. Another reason why I want to try this peptide!

Dr. Pace and I hope you enjoyed the peptide discussion! Thank you to Dr. Pace for allowing me to chime in here on the peptide discussion as it has been an honor. Again, in my personal feeling, this class of products will slowly over time be replacing pharmaceutical compounds for the treatment of many disease states. Please let me know how they worked for you and what combinations you have tried. The VDP will be a living document, and will be updated with your results in volume 2! Please send us your story on Instagram as well!

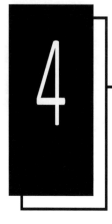

High-Intensity Interval Resistance Training (HIIRT)

D
r. Pace here - thank you, Chris, for the peptide section! This section of the book is critically important! It is a form of exercise that Chris and I do regularly, and I prescribe it to my patients daily. I am sure there are books out there on this alone, as it is a great form of fat-burning exercise. If HIIRT is not possible or it is just not something that excites you as a form of exercise, you still need to move. Sitting on the couch, drinking beer, while doing the rest of the VDP is not going to cut it! Get with your doctor and get on a plan to get your body moving. Start with walking in one direction away from your house for 15 minutes and turn around and walk back home and build up from there. I realize that people reading this book are everything from the morbidly obese to

the marathon runners so HIIRT may not be your thing, but I do love it. Like I have mentioned, the VDP is going to be a living document with volume 2 in the works. In Volume 2, you won't hear from Chris or I much. My goal is to find professionals out there to chime in on these subjects to enrich you, the reader, on your knowledge of all that is presented here in the VDP.

In the spirit of volume 2 of the VDP, I would like to introduce to you, say, our guest speaker, Benton Maslyk. Otherwise known as "Blaze" in the fitness world. Blaze has taught over 6000 HIIRT classes and has been Chris' coach on and off for over 6 years. Blaze is a fitness trainer with the International Sports Sciences Association and has a degree in exercise, sports, and fitness management from Columbus State, OH. Blaze is charismatic and full of energy as I am sure you will feel it here in a moment. Please visit our YouTube channel to meet Blaze in person. Take it away Blaze!

Wow! Thank you, Dr. Pace, for allowing me this honor! let's unpack this and get right to it. HIIRT is about spiking your heart rate and getting your heart rate into a max fat burning zone or getting your heartbeat above 80% of your max heart rate and maintaining that for a few minutes. For Chris, this is

147 beats per minute, though yours will be different. This can be done through floor exercises, stationary bike, the treadmill just to name a few. To get your heart rate up for a longer time, the treadmill or running outside is the best option. Let's look at the word interval. Again, exactly how it sounds, you want to spike your heart rate, then you want to bring it down, spike it, and bring it down. This, in my opinion, is the best fat burning form of exercise. Let's look at resistance. Again, exactly what it says - you have to lift weights if you want them to grow and gain strength. Oh, by the way, ladies with the VDP you are not going to turn into a manly figure or get large muscles! Nothing in the VDP is geared toward bodybuilding so it's OK. Perhaps if you are a competitive bodybuilder in the bikini or figure class the VDP could have a utility. I know Chris' strength and muscle size and definition has certainly improved on the VDP. He has made a concerted effort to lift heavier as he progresses. He started curling 25-pound barbells a year ago, and now 40s are no problem. Yes, I do push him when he is in my class! I don't want to scare you away if you are a gymaphobe, (did I just make up a new word?) but if you are looking for results beyond fat loss you need to lift weights. The VDP and HIIRT is going to give you the energy to do so! It has turned a 53-year-old (Chris) into a 25-year-old

on the inside and made this possible. Before this I just did not think you could build muscle over 40 - I was wrong! Even with all my training in the fitness arena. When I met Chris, he said he was clueless in the gym! He had no idea how to lift weights and he, like many could not afford a personal trainer so I suggested a class type of environment for HIIRT. Whatever form of exercise you and your doctor agree on is good with me. Now let's look at some of the facts behind this and see how I have applied these to Chris's situation. While reading the following points, think of how you can relate to your personal situation. HIIRT and the VDP can be done by the obese and world-class athletes as well.

HIIRT allows you to burn about the same number of calories, but spend less time exercising. This alone was great for Chris and anyone that works full time, has kids, etc. Think about your schedule and getting in an hour a day for 4 to 6 days a week. HIIRT was also found to shift the body's metabolism toward using fat for energy rather than carbs. I am also a fan of intermittent fasting and the low carb keto lifestyle. If you can do your HIIRT routine while fasting or with just protein in your system, I believe you will get better results. I also agree with Dr. Pace big time here - check with your doctor first!

HIIRT is well studied. This is not something that Dr. Pace or I
have invented, and Dr. Pace asked not to make this a scientific
reference manual. With that being said, I do recall one study
found that people performing HIIRT three times per week for
20 minutes per session lost 4.4 pounds, of body fat in 12 weeks
— without any dietary changes, perhaps more important was
the 17% reduction in visceral fat, or the disease-promoting fat
surrounding your internal organs. I believe "the proof is in the
pudding" here if you just look at Chris' before and after pictures concerning the fat loss.

In addition to helping with fat loss, HIIRT could help increase
muscle mass in certain individuals. This is a cornerstone
that Dr. Pace has laid out here in the VPD. I must admit, the
thought of gaining muscle over say 40 or 50 was a stretch for
me. After seeing Chris' gains and the synergy with HIIRT, I am
a believer.

Another study found that eight weeks of HIIRT on a stationary
bike decreased blood pressure as much as traditional continuous endurance training in adults with high blood pressure. I
am a big fan of the stationary bike and cycling classes as well.
Chris prefers the treadmill. The take-home message here is

just to spike your heart rate by any means, elliptical trainer, stair master, running outside - whatever it takes or whatever you enjoy!

In closing, find something you like to do - volleyball, basket-ball, golf (not riding in a cart sipping vodka all day!), swim-ming, yoga, water aerobics, a HIIRT class - just move! I am obviously a huge fan of HIIRT, but I am a bigger fan of just getting you moving. When Dr. Pace asked me to write this section, I was relieved to understand that this is an evi-dence-based protocol as HIIRT is evidence-based as well. It just makes perfect sense to incorporate HIIRT into the VDP. I cannot thank Dr. Pace enough to allowing me on this stage! Looks like Dr. Pace is going to discuss one of my favorite top-ics as well - intermittent fasting.

5

Intermittent Fasting (IF)

T hank you Blaze! Dr. Pace here...HIIRT is so important as it is my form of exercise. I believe when you combine IF with HIIRT, the results can be magnified. Before we get started - like everything in the VDP - check with your doctor on this one as well. IF can be perceived as a little extreme - especially working out while fasting as Chris does. I'll give you the spoiler alert - just eat in an 8-hour window and do not eat for 16 hours. Another really simple way to look at this is to skip breakfast. Oh boy, there is another can of worms! All the breakfast eating gurus are coming unglued right now! Then again, all the intermittent fasting people are clapping their hands. In my personal opinion, if you need to lose weight or have any type of metabolic disorder breakfast is the worst meal of the day. The thought of a bowl of cereal, a few pieces of toast with jelly first thing in the morning makes my blood boil and will send your insulin through the roof and adds to you packing on the pounds.

Let's talk through this for a second. Your liver stores glycogen for energy. Glycogen is a form of energy we get from our diet. If you don't use that energy, it turns into fat. I have Chris work out in the morning on an empty stomach, just black coffee. Therefore, he is using up his glycogen stores for energy thus preventing them from turning into fat. When you are in a fasting state, your body is in repair mode. Your body is also mobilizing fat to be used for energy. As soon as you put food in your stomach bells and whistles go off inside your body. They turn every energetic metabolic process to your stomach and your intestines to digest the food. Insulin is elevated, and this causes excess calories to be stored in your fat cells. We could do a deeper clinical dive here, but I just hope this tidbit makes since.

What I do know is Chris' cholesterol levels have normalized and I feel that IF has a lot to do with it. How does Chris break his fast? He has a dark berry and greens superfoods protein smoothie at about 10:30 am. I am a big fan of superfoods and we can discuss more in that chapter. So, in that case, his eating window is 8 hours from 10:30 am to 6:30 pm. If happy hour lasts till 7:00 pm then he may stretch it a bit and have a later dinner. In that case he will extend the window of eating out further the next day.

There are a few more ways to do IF. Get with your doctor and get a plan that works for you. Another type is known as 5:2. or simply no or little food for two days out of the week. Some say eat 500-600 calories on those two days and spread out the days to say like Tuesday and Thursdays as your fasting days.

Another similar concept would be to fast for 24 hours once or twice a week. One way to think about this would be to have dinner, then don't eat until dinner the next evening. This is known in some circles as the eat-stop-eat fast. Some say eat breakfast, then don't eat until breakfast the next day. For me, maybe it's psychological, I would just like to go to bed with a little food in me and go from dinner to dinner. Again, whatever works with you and your doctor.

Another not so popular form that you may hear about is alternate day fasting. For me, this would not be fun, but it may work for you. Just the concept of going to bed hungry does nothing for me. Keep in mind that in the morning I am in the Cath lab and my mind is super focused on my procedures, so food is not at the top of my mind. Your schedule may be right for this, so it was worthy of mentioning.

Then there is a concept known as warrior dieting. This is basically eating dinner only. Some say snack fruits and veggies during the day. This came out of the paleo movement which I will cover more in the diet chapter of this book. This concept seems doable again depends on your schedule etc.

The last concept may be right for you. Just skipping meals randomly. Think about our ancestors. They did not pull into McDonald's three times a day to eat. Find one of these IF methods that work for you. If you have a pre-existing eating disorder, none of these may be the thing for you. Chris is openly a food addict and has a black and white personality with the absence of a throttle. Only an on-off switch. Therefore the 16/8 method works best for Chris and I. Like most of the concepts in the VDP, this is a personalized approach. Your dose of hormones, choice of peptide, diet, etc. is all meant to be personalized to your body, situation, and goals. The type of IF fasting should fit into your lifestyle and hopefully agreed upon with your doctor. One more idea is to do a cleansing fast or a 24-hour juice fast of celery, spinach, kale, and apple, etc. Chris does this a few times a year.

Let's wrap this up and mention the benefits of IF. This sums up all the forms of IF we mentioned.

- Insulin levels: Blood levels of insulin drop significantly, which facilitates fat burning.
- Human growth hormone: The blood levels of growth hormone may increase as much as 5-fold - way cool on the VDP!
- Cellular repair: The body induces important cellular repair processes, such as removing waste material from cells
- Gene expression: There are beneficial changes in several genes and molecules related to longevity and protection against disease
- Enhances hormone function to facilitate weight loss - has been shown to have major benefits for insulin resistance and lead to an impressive reduction in blood sugar levels
- Studies show that IF can help fight inflammation, another key driver of all sorts of common diseases

- Has been shown to improve numerous different risk factors, including blood pressure, total and LDL cholesterol, blood triglycerides, inflammatory markers, and blood sugar levels as Chris has proven.

- Increases autophagy (removing waste from cells) may provide protection against several diseases, including cancer and Alzheimer's disease

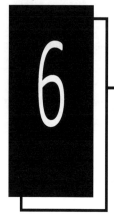

chapter

Supplements/ Nutraceuticals

H i, Dr. Pace here again to discuss supplements or nutraceuticals, also known as nutras. In today's food supply we are so depleted of nutrients. Just about everything has been genetically modified, and we do not get the nutrition we need and that our bodies are craving. Just like everything in the VDP, there is a point and a counterpoint, same with nutras! There is a camp that says all nutras are a waste of money. I can kind of see their point as it relates purely to the weight loss industry. Do you need to take a nutra to lose weight? No. Keep in mind though that the VDP is not purely a weight loss program, yet a body transformation and longevity program. Therefore, I feel this discussion is valid here. As we have learned, Chris is a little OCD on the VDP and nutras, so I will point out what I feel is particularly relevant to the core VDP while keeping your wallet in mind. Let's cover some big ones and then we can dive into some clinical pearls as well. These are not discussed in any particular order, or order of importance. I guess the big one if you are on BHRT would be DIM, so perk up in that section below. I am also a big fan of the data surrounding Vitamin D. I encourage you to research these further as, again, books could be and are written on these individual nutras.

Probiotics

The flora, the bacteria, or the microbiome in your stomach and intestinal tract is the gateway and the building blocks to your immune system. Immune cells are produced here and exist from your throat to your large colon. All these bacteria are what we call symbiotic or living together. I have done extensive research into biofilm which could be another book in itself but I will try to stay on track here! Also, these cells are intelligent little creatures, and they do communicate with each other through a system called quorum sensing - amazing stuff!

Anyway, after a course of antibiotics or a nice GMO laden meal, this gut bacteria or flora gets destroyed or greatly disrupted. Therefore, a daily good high grade 4 or 5 billion species probiotic is critical. Make sure you get a good, reputable brand. I am also a believer in kombucha, and it has a nice caloric profile for the VDP.

Probiotics are live microorganisms that are intended to have health benefits. Products sold as probiotics include foods (such as yogurt), dietary supplements, and products that aren't used orally, such as skin creams. Both Chris and I take a probiotic every day usually in the morning on an empty stomach. I encourage you to do more research in this area as you can write an entire book on the gut bacterial microbiome. In a nutshell, there are friendly bacteria that exist from your throat all the way to your colon. These bacteria are the foundation for every immune response we have in our bodies. Probiotics keep this "flora" in balance, and it has a profound downstream effect on your immune system, metabolism, and disease prevention. People often think of bacteria and other microorganisms as harmful "germs," many microorganisms help our bodies function properly. For example, bacteria that are normally present in our intestines help digest food, destroy disease-causing microorganisms, and produce vitamins. Large numbers of microorganisms live on and in our bodies. Many of the microorganisms in probiotic products are the same as or like microorganisms that naturally live in our bodies. Probiotics may contain a variety of microorganisms. The most common are bacteria that belong to groups called Lactobacillus and Bifidobacterium. Each of these two broad groups includes many types of bacteria. Other bacteria may also be used as probiotics and yeast such as Saccharomyces boulardii. Researchers have studied probiotics to find out whether they might help prevent or treat a variety of health problems, including:

- Digestive disorders such as diarrhea caused by infections, antibiotic-associated diarrhea, irritable bowel syndrome, and inflammatory bowel disease
- Allergic disorders such as atopic dermatitis (eczema) and allergic rhinitis (hay fever)
- Tooth decay, periodontal disease, and other oral health problems
- Colic in infants
- Liver disease
- The common cold
- Prevention of necrotizing enterocolitis in very low birth weight infants.

There's preliminary evidence that some probiotics are helpful in preventing diarrhea caused by infections and antibiotics and in improving symptoms of irritable bowel syndrome, but more needs to be learned. We still don't know which probiotics are helpful and which are not. We also don't know how much of the probiotic people would have to take or who would most likely benefit from taking probiotics. Even for the conditions that have been studied the most, researchers are still working toward finding the answers to these questions.

Probiotics are not alike. Make sure you get a good one from a reputable manufacturer. For example, if a specific kind of Lactobacillus helps prevent an illness, that doesn't necessarily mean that another kind of Lactobacillus would have the same effect or that any of the Bifidobacterium probiotics would do the same thing. Although some probiotics have shown promise in research studies, strong scientific evidence to support specific uses of probiotics for most health conditions is lacking.

I was going to write a chapter on GMO (genetically modified organisms) foods, Monsanto corporation, and organic farming and nutrition. After consideration and keeping to the VDP, I realized that you can have the same success with the VDP eating conventional foods. This is taking into the fact that you are doing the VDP for body composition and not, say cancer prevention. I did want to mention this as Chris, and I do try to eat organic when possible, and I try to eat grass-fed, organically raised and free-range beef and chicken when possible as well. I am also surprised at the number of patients I have that are not aware of GMO foods, Monsanto corporation and the evils of roundup weed killer. These all have a negative effect on our microbiome, so let's have a quick discussion here in the probiotic section.

In a nutshell, Monsanto corporation has developed a way to genetically modify crops, mostly corn and soy to be round up resistant. Round up is the popular weed killer manufactured by Monsanto and is currently in the news with the cancer lawsuits. The GMO corn and soy are grown by large commercial farms. The farmers can spray roundup on the crops, and it kills all the weeds surrounding the corn and soy, and the corn and soy survive. This concept alone should be alarming as we are putting this crop in our bodies. Monsanto sells these seeds to farmers and 92% of the corn we eat is GMO now.

Why have you not heard of this? Labeling laws and government corruption. We have laws in this country that allow GMO foods to be sold without GMO labeling. In Europe and most industrialized nations, GMO labeling is required and GMO crops are becoming banned. Please do some research and perhaps I will do a YouTube video on this so you can have more information and some resources on this.

Let's take a little dive into what these foods do to our microbiome and why a probiotic is a good idea. Round up also known as glycophosphate. Preliminary studies are showing the effect of glyphosate on gut bacteria. This research is still limited since the impact of herbicides like glyphosate on gut health is chronic in nature (versus acute), with believed symptoms and changes to microbiota evolving with long-term consistent exposure. Therefore, much of the research just needs more time.

That said, researchers looking at gastrointestinal (GI) bacteria in chickens found that beneficial bacteria were more susceptible to the pesticide and harmful bacteria more resistant, when exposed to high levels. Additionally, we've seen studies linking glyphosate as a causal factor in the rise of both gluten intolerance and celiac disease, both of which are intricately inter-twined with the health of our gut and makeup of microbiota. This is important to know as gluten is seen as the culprit here. Perhaps we should take another look. Hopefully, in volume 2, I will have an expert submit something in this area, remember I am a cardiologist, not a nutritionist. Also, we have studies today that show how glyphosate interferes with a specific bio-chemical pathway involved with the synthesis of amino acid proteins and while this pathway is not found in humans, it is a pathway found in the bacteria in the gastrointestinal (GI) tract. Therefore, when exposed, glyphosate inhibits the growth of any beneficial bacteria in the gut, resulting in the need for a probiotic.

I hope that did not sound like a political rant, I just felt it is an area of health and our food supply that you should be aware of. Just pay more attention to your labels, do your research and hopefully, you will find a good probiotic and restore your gut health.

Vitamin D

Let's face it. We as Americans are so scared of the sun that when we go out in the sun, we are covered with 70 SPF sunscreen, so quite frankly we're just not getting enough vitamin D. Now all my dermatology friends are yelling at me. My wish is that in volume 2 we have a dermatologist chime in here as SPF, the sun and Vitamin D is a hot topic. We're certainly are not getting vitamin D from the GMO foods we eat.

More than likely you've never had your vitamin D level checked. Most of my patients have baseline levels around 20. You want your D level over 60. Again, this is not a scientific reference book or manual, but the data shows that your chance of getting cancer is lowered at a Vitamin D level of over 60. This is another can of worms as when one study shows vitamin D reduces cancer, another says it has no effect. An important thing to consider is the proper combination of vitamins with vitamin D and the form of vitamin D. The critical thing is that you need to combine D3 with vitamin A and vitamin K2. The absorption of vitamin D3 in this combination also works synergistically with your hormone pellets to increase bone mineral density and to make strong bones.

This is a serious area for your health, so let's look at this a little deeper. Vitamin D helps the body to use calcium and phosphorus for strong bones and teeth. Skin exposed to sunshine can make vitamin D, and vitamin D can also be obtained from certain foods. Vitamin D deficiency can cause a weakening of the bones (which is rickets in children and osteomalacia in adults). Dietary sources include a few foods that naturally contain vitamin D, such as fatty fish, fish liver oil, and eggs, sorry Chris! However, most dietary vitamin D comes from foods fortified with vitamin D, such as milk, juices, and breakfast cereals. Vitamin D can also be obtained through dietary supplements. Therefore, vegan Chris takes his A, D, K supplement!

Make sure you check with your doctor on the amount to take. Even though most people are unlikely to have high vitamin D intakes, it is important to remember that excessive intake of any nutrient, including vitamin D, can cause toxic effects. Too much vitamin D can be harmful because it increases calcium levels.

A little more on the sun and vitamin D. Excessive sun exposure does not cause vitamin D toxicity. However, people should not try to increase vitamin D production by increasing their exposure to sunlight because this will also increase their risk of skin cancer. So being a Floridian - this is cool - early epidemiologic research showed that incidence and death rates for certain cancers were lower among individuals living in southern latitudes, where levels of sunlight exposure are relatively higher than among those living at northern latitudes. Because exposure to ultraviolet light from sunlight leads to the production of vitamin D, researchers hypothesize that variation in vitamin D levels might account for this association. However, additional research is required to determine whether higher vitamin D levels are related to lower cancer incidence or death rates. I am careful not to burn in the sun, but I do get deliberate sun, just enough to maintain some color and I also take a vitamin A, D, K supplement daily. This is another request of any colleagues out there to please contribute to Volume 2 of the VDP in the area of vitamin D.

B Vitamins

Methylation - let's start here with a big word! I am trying to keep this book as educational as possible but sometimes we need to look a little deeper at some things - so let's go! Make sure your B vitamins are methylated - why? Because it's widely understood that a certain percentage (possibly as high as 60%) of the population are unable to metabolize the unmethylated forms of specific B vitamins, namely folate and vitamin B12. This is a big deal! Genetic testing has become increasingly more accessible to the public for identifying carriers of one (or both) of the genetic abnormalities, C677t and A1298c, that prevent the metabolism of unmethylated forms of B vitamins. For that, it's easy to see why an increasing number of consumers are now concerned with methylation.

Think of methylation, and the opposite action, demethylation, as the mechanism that allows the gears to turn, and turns biological switches on and off for a host of systems in the body. You want a good mixture of B12, B6, and folic acid. These are critical for homocysteine levels as they will lower homocysteine levels. Homocysteine has been tied to increase cardiovascular

91

events. As a part of the VDP, your doctor may or may not get a homocysteine level. I checked Chris' and he was high before starting the VDP, 20 was his level. After taking a methylated B complex it was cut in half in 3 months down to a level of 9. This is perhaps not critical to the VDP concerning weight loss and body composition, but I just wanted to share the experience that Chris had with homocysteine. Proper methylation influences so many systems in our bodies that it often gets overlooked, which can severely impact how well your body functions. Ask your health-care practitioner for advice if you have any concerns about the methylation of homocysteine. I don't get too wrapped up with homocysteine and heart disease, but it is a piece of the inflammatory puzzle and worthy of a discussion with your doctor.

DIM - Diindolymethane

DIM is a big one! We could write a book on this alone! DIM is a must if you're on hormone pellets as DIM helps metabolize, in both men and women, hormone pellets down the correct metabolic pathway. Women should take your DIM once a day and men take it two times a day or as directed by your doctor.

DIM is extracts of cruciferous vegetables mostly broccoli and kale. Men, DIM is an absolute must while on hormone therapy as it can also aid in preventing from aromatizing testosterone, we discussed that in the section under testosterone. Ladies, DIM will also encourage estrogen to break down into the 'good' metabolites rather than the 'bad' ones." This "good" estrogen is thought to have a protective effect against breast cancer. So basically, it's helpful for hormonal imbalances.

Chris had an interesting experience with DIM. His first round of BHRT pellets his testosterone was 1384 and his estradiol was 57 at his one-month checkup and blood test. This is a fine ratio. He was taking his DIM and felt great. On his second round, we decided to go down a tad on his testosterone pellets. He reported feeling not as good as the first round. His testosterone was at 985 and his estradiol was 101. This is too high of an estradiol level for a man. Well, Chris can be a little stubborn and he stopped taking the DIM that I and his primary hormone doctor recommended. He admitted to taking some products he ordered online. We all learned a lesson here - make sure you have a high-quality DIM!

I also want to take a second and thank Chris' doctor that does his insertions, Dr. Tami Horner. We have collaborated on Chris' care and she has been a source of knowledge and has helped mentor me in this process. A big thank you, Dr. Horner! Hopefully, she will help with volume 2 as she is a notable thought leader in the area of BHRT. On Chris' 3rd. round, his testosterone level was 1114 and his estradiol level was 47 - perfection! Short story? Take your DIM!

Now back to the ladies - in addition to taking DIM on BHRT, I recommend DIM for women who are showing symptoms of estrogen dominance, which often include heavy periods, periods longer than seven days, menstrual cycles shorter than 25 days, and emotional PMS symptoms—major mood swings, irritability, uncontrollable anger, and feelings of depression. Some women report seeing improvement after only a few doses, whereas others need to take it for three to four weeks before seeing noticeable changes. Also, I need to acknowledge and thank my wife. Dr. Michelle Lemay, OBGYN. She has been a big resource and helps in treating the ladies in my practice. Without her, I would have a tough time here. Some days I burden her with texts concerning women and BHRT. I want to thank her and tell her how much I love her and hopefully, she will have a big role in volume 2 of the VDP.

Another item we need to discuss is sex hormone-binding globulin or SHBG. Again, you can write a book on SHBG. There is a relationship between SHBG and DIM, so I thought we could discuss it here. This is true for men and women. Testosterone acts differently depending on whether it is free or bound to carrier proteins in the blood, or SHBG. DIM, through its effects on estrogen metabolism, supports testosterone by helping to maintain the level of free or active testosterone. Free testosterone refers to the diffraction of testosterone that circulates in the blood and is not associated with or bound by SHBG, its carrier protein. Since only free testosterone easily crosses into the brain, muscles, and fat cells much of the desirable action of testosterone has to do with the free portion. However, this represents only a tiny amount of the total testosterone equal to only 2% of the total in men and even less in women. Remember we discussed how good your mood is on BHRT? That is part of the reason. High levels of SHBG lock-up free testosterone making it unavailable to support mood or metabolism. Interestingly, unmetabolized estrogen is the body's primary signal to increase the production and levels of the testosterone-binding protein. Low levels of free testosterone have been identified during perimenopause and are most dramatic in women with severe premenstrual syndrome (PMS) symptoms. Birth control pills also cause high SHBG.

Since DIM promotes a more active metabolism of estrogen, un-metabolized estrogen levels fall and the 2-hydroxy-estrogens increase. The 2-hydroxy-estrogens possess the unique ability to displace testosterone from SHGB and set it free. Therefore, the combined effect of DIM to reduce unmetabolized estrogen and increase 2-hydroxy-estrogens can reduce elevations in SHGB and allow for freer testosterone. Both changes help maintain and restore a youthful balance between estrogen and free testosterone. This balance is key to healthy and active metabolism and feeling great on the VDP. I mention all this as it is it can be an area of discussion with your doctor. I and your doctor want you to get the most benefit from the VDP, SHBG, and DIM could be a part of the puzzle in your VDP life.

One more closing thought for men and DIM. Taking DIM has resulted in reports of improved prostate function based on reduced nighttime urination in symptomatic older men. As we said, DIM is uniquely active in promoting healthy estrogen metabolism and improving symptoms of estrogen-related imbalance. Even more impressive is research showing that unmetabolized estrogen accumulates in prostate tissue in men as they age. Exposure of human prostate tissue to unmetabolized estrogen in the laboratory did indeed result in activation and increased the production of prostate-specific antigen protein (PSA). Men, check with your doctor on PSA levels and BHRT. The PSA protein level in men's blood is now used as a screening test to determine the severity of prostate enlargement or to determine the chance of prostate cancer. Recent studies also have shown that estradiol, the active form of estrogen, causes the prostate gland to increase its production of PSA. Increased PSA production, however, can be inhibited by the "good" estrogen metabolites promoted by DIM. This indicates that "good" estrogen metabolites are more beneficial for prostate health than unmetabolized estrogen-like estradiol. The optimal testosterone-to-estrogen hormonal balance achieved with the use of DIM can help to preserve a youthful urinary tract, prevent age-related prostate growth, and perhaps reduce the risk of prostate cancer. This is nice to close DIM with as that statement sort of sums up the VDP. Optimal and balance are the cornerstone of the VDP.

L-Arginine
L-Citrulline Complex

Here is another one that Chris takes, usually before his HIIRT. These two are wonderful when taken together and can be a great adjunct in the area of nitric oxide (NO) production. NO has a profound impact on vasodilation and vasoconstriction in your vessels and has a good effect on your blood pressure as well. Hence the cardiologist in me perks up! Let me bullet point some of the effects.

- Supports muscle metabolism, energy, heart function, and circulation
- Supports liver detoxification and both are key intermediates in the Krebs urea cycle, where they participate in the detoxification of ammonia via the production of urea
- The formation of NO mediates smooth muscle relaxation in the blood vessel wall, and thus reduces the workload of the heart
- Many nerve cells also use NO as a signaling molecule, erectile function, for example, is mediated by the release of NO.
- Also, l-Arginine is an important factor in muscle metabolism promoting energy during exercise and increased recovery after a workout

We could spend more time here as the Nobel peace prize was awarded in 1998 to the researchers that discovered NO in the arteries. A popular blood pressure medication class - ace inhibitors use a similar mechanism of action.

Iodine

We mentioned this in the thyroid section a few chapters back. It is critical to thyroid function so very worthy of some time spent here on this mineral. Thyroid hormones play an important role in a wide range of bodily functions, including metabolism, bone health, immune response, and development of the central nervous system (CNS). Iodine helps convert thyroid-stimulating hormone (TSH) to triiodothyronine (T3) and thyroxine (T4). Remember the T3, T4 discussion? This conversion is important for the thyroid to function properly.

An iodine imbalance can lead to an overactive or underactive thyroid. Around 70 to 80 percent of iodine is found in the thyroid gland in the neck. The rest is in the blood, the muscles, the ovaries, and other parts of the body. An estimated 2 billion people worldwide remain at risk for iodine deficiency, and about 300 million people worldwide suffer from thyroid gland dysfunction.

Let me bullet point some key facts about iodine:

- Iodine is an important nutrient for thyroid functioning.
- Too much iodine or too little iodine can lead to symptoms of hyperthyroidism or hypothyroidism.
- Good sources of iodine are seaweed and iodized salt or by supplementation.

Iodine deficiency is rare in western countries, and additional iodine should only be taken with a doctor's supervision.

That sums up our nutra discussion. Are all these critical to the VDP? No, they are all worthy of discussion and should lead to individual discussions with your doctor. Remember DIM is the big one if on BHRT. Now let's go and open the biggest can of worms in the VDP!

Diet

O
h boy!! This will be fun! I think in volume 2, I will turn this section over to my colleagues. Before we get started, I want to reiterate, again, that contradictory to its name, the VDP is not a diet. Just a fun catchy name that does include diet as part of the protocol. I will not tell you what to eat here. Chris and I will lay out some ideas for you and tell Chris' story. Before we start our discussion just look at some diets out there:

- Cookie diet: A calorie control diet in which low-fat cookies are eaten to quell hunger, often in place of a meal.

- The Hacker's Diet: A calorie-control diet from *The Hacker's Diet* by John Walker. The book suggests that the key to reaching and maintaining the desired weight is understanding and carefully monitoring calories consumed and used.

- Nutrisystem diet: The dietary element of the weight-loss plan from Nutrisystem, Inc. Nutrisystem distributes low-calorie meals, with specific ratios of fats, proteins, and carbohydrates.

- Weight Watchers diet: Foods are assigned point values; dieters can eat any food with a point value provided they stay within their daily point limit.

- A very low-calorie diet is consuming fewer than 800 calories per day. Such diets are normally followed under the supervision of a doctor. Zero-calorie diets are also included.

- India (breatharian diet): A diet in which no food is consumed, based on the belief that food is not necessary for human subsistence.

- KE diet: A diet in which an individual feeds through a feeding tube and does not eat anything.

- Atkins diet: A low-carbohydrate diet, popularized by nutritionist Robert Atkins in the late-20th and early-21st centuries. Proponents argue that this approach is a more successful way of losing weight than low-calorie diets, critics argue that a low-carb approach poses increased health risks. The Atkins diet consists of four phases (Induction, Balancing,

Fine-Tuning, and Maintenance) with a gradual increase in the consumption of carbohydrates as the person goes through the phases.

- Dukan Diet: A multi-step diet based on high protein and limited carbohydrate consumption. It starts with two steps intended to facilitate short term weight loss, followed by two steps intended to consolidate these losses and return to a more balanced long-term diet.

- Kimkins: A heavily promoted diet for weight loss, found to be fraudulent.

- South Beach Diet: Diet developed by the Miami-based cardiologist Arthur Agatston, M.D., who says that the key to losing weight quickly and getting healthy isn't cutting all carbohydrates and fats from your diet but choosing the right carbs and the right fats.

- Stillman diet: A carbohydrate-restricted diet that predates the Atkins diet, allowing consumption of specific food ingredients.

- McDougall's starch diet is a high calorie, high fiber, low-fat diet that is based on starches such as potatoes, rice, and beans which excludes all animal foods and added vegetable oils. John A. McDougall draws on historical observation of how many civilizations around the world throughout time have thrived on starch foods.

- Beverly Hills Diet: An extreme diet that has only fruits in the first days, gradually increasing the selection of foods up to the sixth week.

- Cabbage soup diet: A low-calorie diet based on heavy consumption of cabbage soup. Considered a fad diet.

- Grapefruit diet: A fad diet, intended to facilitate weight loss, in which grapefruit is consumed in large quantities at mealtimes.

- Monotropic diet: A diet that involves eating only one food item, or one type of food, for a period of time to achieve a desired weight reduction.

- Subway diet: A crash diet in which a person consumes Subway sandwiches in place of higher-calorie fast foods. Made famous by a former obese student, who lost 245 pounds after replacing his meals with Subway sandwiches as part of an effort to lose weight.

- Western dietary pattern: A diet consisting of food which is most commonly consumed in developed countries. Examples include meat, white bread, milk, and puddings. The name is a reference to the Western world.

- Juice fasting: A form of a detox diet, in which nutrition is obtained solely from fruit and vegetable juices. The health implications of such diets are disputed.

- Master Cleanse: A form of juice fasting.
- The DASH diet (Dietary Approaches to Stop Hypertension): A recommendation that those with high blood pressure consume large quantities of fruits, vegetables, whole-grains, and low-fat dairy foods as part of their diet, and avoid sugar-sweetened foods, red meat, and fats. Promoted by the US Department of Health and Human Services, a United States government organization.
- Diabetic diet: An umbrella term for diets recommended to people with diabetes. There is considerable disagreement in the scientific community as to what sort of diet is best for people with diabetes.
- Elemental diet: A medical, liquid-only diet, in which liquid nutrients are consumed for ease of ingestion.
- Elimination diet: A method of identifying foods which cause a person adverse effects, by process of elimination.
- Gluten-free diet: A diet that avoids the protein gluten, which is found in barley, rye, and wheat. It is a medical treatment for gluten-related disorders, which include coeliac disease, non-celiac gluten sensitivity, gluten ataxia, dermatitis herpetiformis and wheat allergy.
  - Gluten-free, casein-free diet: A gluten-free diet which also avoids casein, a protein commonly found in milk and

cheese. This diet has been researched for efficacy in the treatment of autism spectrum disorder.

- Healthy kidney diet: This diet is for those impacted with chronic kidney disease, those with only one kidney who have a kidney infection and those who may be suffering from some other kidney failure. This diet is not the dialysis diet, which is something completely different. The healthy kidney diet restricts large amounts of protein which are hard for the kidney to break down but especially limits: potassium and phosphorus-rich foods and beverages. Liquids are often restricted as well—not forbidden, just less of.

  - Ketogenic diet: A high-fat, low-carb diet, in which dietary and body fat is converted into energy. It is used as a medical treatment for refractory epilepsy.

  - Liquid diet: A diet in which only liquids are consumed. May be administered by clinicians for medical reasons, such as after a gastric bypass or to prevent death through starvation from a hunger strike.

  - Low-FODMAP diet: A diet that consists of the global restriction of all fermentable carbohydrates (FODMAPs).

  - Soft diet

  - Specific carbohydrate diet: A diet that aims to restrict the intake of complex carbohydrates such as found in grains and complex sugars. It is promoted as a way of reducing the symptoms of irritable bowel syndrome (IBS), Crohn's disease, ulcerative colitis, coeliac disease, and autism.

- Alkaline diet
- Baby Food Diet
- Cabbage soup diet
- Food combining diet: A nutritional approach where certain food types are deliberately consumed together or separately. For instance, some weight control diets suggest that proteins and carbohydrates should not be consumed in the same meal.
  - Fit for Life diet: Recommendations include not combining protein and carbohydrates, not drinking water at mealtime, and avoiding dairy foods.
- Fruitarianism
- Gluten-free diet, while essential for people with celiac disease or gluten sensitivity, has also become a fad.
- Grapefruit diet
- Lambchop and pineapple diet
- Morning banana diet
- Superfood diet
- Whole30 diet
- Dukan Diet

- Low-carbohydrate diet
  - Atkins diet
  - "Keto" or ketogenic diet (but for the purpose of weight loss instead of epilepsy seizures reduction)
  - Salisbury diet
  - Stillman diet
  - Sugar Busters
  - Zone diet: A diet in which a person attempts to split calorie intake from carbohydrates, proteins, and fats in a 40:30:30 ratio.
  - Other high-fat variants.
- Paleolithic diet: Can refer either to the eating habits of humans during the Paleolithic era or of modern dietary plans purporting to be based on these habits.
- Scarsdale medical diet
- South Beach Diet
- The 4-Hour Body
- Liquid diets
  - Cambridge Diet
  - Slim-Fast
- KE diet
- Juice fasting
- Detox diet

- Lemon detox diet
- Breatharian diet: A diet based on a belief that people can sustain with spirituality and sunlight alone but leads to starvation and devotees have been spotted eating and drinking in hiding.
- Blood type diet: A diet based on a belief that people's diets should reflect their blood types.
- High carb/low-fat diets
  - Dr. Dean Ornish: Eat More, Weigh Less
  - The Good Carbohydrate Revolution
  - The Pritikin Principle or Pritikin Program for Diet and Exercise or Pritikin Diet: A diet which focusses on the consumption of unprocessed food.
- Immune Power Diet
- Macrobiotics
- Fruitarian diet: A diet that predominantly consists of raw fruit.
- Lacto vegetarianism: A vegetarian diet that includes certain types of dairy, but excludes eggs and foods which contain animal rennet. A common diet among followers of several religions, including Hinduism, Sikhism, and Jainism, based on the principle of Ahimsa (non-harming).
- Ova vegetarianism: A vegetarian diet that includes eggs but excludes dairy.

- Ovo-Lacto vegetarianism: A vegetarian diet that includes eggs and dairy.

- Vegan diet: In addition to the abstentions of a vegetarian diet, vegans do not use any product produced by animals, such as eggs, dairy products, or honey. The vegan philosophy and lifestyle is broader than just the diet and also includes abstaining from using any products tested on animals and often campaigning for animal rights

- Semi-vegetarianism: A predominantly vegetarian diet, in which meat is occasionally consumed.

- Kangatarian: A diet originating from Australia. In addition to foods permissible in a vegetarian diet, kangaroo meat is also consumed.

- Pescatarian diet: A diet that includes fish but no other meats.

- Plant-based diet: A broad term to describe diets in which animal products do not form a large proportion of the diet. Under some definitions a plant-based diet is fully vegetarian; under others, it is possible to follow a plant-based diet whilst occasionally consuming meat.

- Pollotarian: Someone who eats chicken or other poultry, but not meat from mammals, often for environmental, health or food justice reasons.

- Pollo-pescatarian: Someone who eats both poultry and fish/seafood, though no meat from mammals

- Alkaline diet: The avoidance of relatively acidic foods – foods with low pH levels – such as alcohol, caffeine, dairy, fungi, grains, meat, and sugar. Proponents believe such a diet may have health benefits;] critics consider the arguments to have no scientific basis.

- Eat-clean diet: Focusses on eating foods without preservatives, and on mixing lean proteins with complex carbohydrates.

- Gerson therapy: A form of alternative medicine, the diet is low salt, low fat, and vegetarian, and also involves taking specific supplements. It was developed by Max Gerson, who claimed the therapy could cure cancer and chronic, degenerative diseases.

- The Graham Diet: A vegetarian diet which promotes whole-wheat flour and discourages the consumption of stimulants such as alcohol and caffeine. Developed by Sylvester Graham in the 19th century.

- Hay diet: A food-combining diet developed by William Howard Hay in the 1920s. Divides foods into separate groups, and suggests that proteins and carbohydrates should not be consumed in the same meal.

- High-protein diet: A diet in which high quantities of protein are consumed with the intention of building muscle. Not to be confused with low-carb diets, where the intention is to lose weight by restricting carbohydrates.

- High residue diet: A diet in which high quantities of dietary fiber are consumed. High-fiber foods include certain fruits, vegetables, nuts, and grains.

- Inuit diet: Inuit people traditionally consume food that is fished, hunted or gathered locally; predominantly meat and fish.

- Jenny Craig: A weight-loss program from Jenny Craig, Inc. It includes weight counseling among other elements. The dietary aspect involves the consumption of pre-packaged food produced by the company.

- Locavore diet: a neologism describing the eating of food that is locally produced, and not moved long distances to market. An example of this was explored in the book 100-Mile Diet, in which the authors only consumed food grown within 100 miles of their residence for a year. People who follow this type of diet are sometimes known as locavores.

- Low carbon diet: Consuming food which has been produced, prepared and transported with a minimum of associated greenhouse gas emissions.

- Low-fat diet

- Low glycemic index diet

- Low-protein diet

- Low sodium diet

- Low-sulfur diet

- Macrobiotic diet: A diet in which processed food is avoided. Common components include grains, beans and vegetables.

- Mediterranean diet: A diet based on the habits of some southern European countries. One of the more distinctive features is that olive oil is used as the primary source of fat.

- MIND diet: combines portions of the DASH diet and the Mediterranean diet. The diet is intended to reduce neurological deterioration such as Alzheimer's disease.

- Montignac diet: A weight-loss diet characterized by consuming carbohydrates with a low glycemic index.

- Negative calorie diet: A claim by many weight-loss diets that some foods take more calories to digest than they provide, such as celery. The basis for this claim is disputed.

- Okinawa diet: A low-calorie diet based on the traditional eating habits of people from the Ryukyu Islands.

- Omnivore: An omnivore consumes both plant and animal-based food.

- Organic food diet: A diet consisting only of food which is organic – it has not been produced with modern inputs such as synthetic fertilizers, genetic modification, irradiation, or synthetic food additives.

- Prison loaf: A meal replacement served in some United States prisons to inmates who are not trusted to use cutlery. Its composition varies between institutions and states, but as a replacement for standard food, it is intended to provide inmates with all their dietary needs.

- Raw foodism: A diet which centers on the consumption of uncooked and unprocessed food. Often associated with a vegetarian diet, although some raw food dieters do consume raw meat.

- Shangri-La Diet

- Slimming World diet

- Slow-carb diet

- Smart for Life

- Sonoma diet: A diet based on portion control and centered around consuming "power foods"

- Spark People diet

- Sugar Busters!: Focuses on restricting the consumption of refined carbohydrates, particularly sugars.

- Tongue Patch Diet: Stitching a Marlex patch to the tongue to make eating painful.

- The Vodka Diet - a revolutionary protocol developed by

a prominent cardiologist utilizing cutting edge technology and incorporating the use of hormones, peptides, and proper nutrition.

OK, that last one I threw in there! Anyway, thank you to my friends from Wikipedia for that shortlist. The take-home message here is that diet can be so confusing and extremely controversial. Another reason why I listed these is, there are many people that have created these diets that have far more training in nutrition than I. I am reaching out to them for participation in volume 2. Oh - do you know how many hours of nutrition training I and most doctors out there receive in medical school? Zero! Just sayin!

Chris and I will take turns here, moving forward in the diet chapter. This is where you will hear a prominent Cardiologist and a hormone/peptide nerd respectfully disagree on a few points, but this will be fun! There are three big points of polarity here, Chris is vegan, I like the Keto diet and Chris loves the HCG diet. One thing we agree on and the takeaway message is to listen to your doctor and lose fat!! Remember that the VDP is a protocol, not a diet. We both agree that a diet is a shorter distance to weight loss. With the VDP I want to develop a healthy lifestyle program for life. let me ask Chris to discuss what he has been up to in the diet world, then I will chime in my success with the keto diet.

Thank you again, Dr. Pace! Let me get the vegan thing behind us. This book is no way trying to get you to go vegan, no agenda here. Just in true transparency, these are the food choices I feel are the best for me. Actually, I am whole foods plant based (WFPB). Let me talk about vegan vs. WFPB. Oreos are vegan! There's so much vegan junk food out there! A vegan way of eating can promote obesity if not eaten the correct way. "Veganism" is almost like a religion or a way of life to protect the environment etc. I do love this planet and do everything possible and teach my daughter everything possible to protect the planet. I just can't throw out a pair of perfect shoes because they are made of animal skin. You get the idea here? My motivation for eating WFPB comes from my Dad's health and a blood test I had about three years ago. Being a chef from Texas, eating a smoker full of BBQ all week for 30 years led to the writing on the wall. I also learned about epigenetics or altering your genetic destination through proper nutrition.

My Dad is alive and well, thank God! He is 77, active, post-heart attack, post-high Gleason prostate cancer, post radical robotic prostatectomy with complications, diabetes and diabetic neuropathy. He is the medical community and the pharmaceutical industry's best client! I would just like to be 77 and have my prostate and no stent in my heart. Again, this is not a vegan agenda, just keeping it real and transparent. If you want more on WFPB, please look up the China study. Oh, vodka is vegan :) Now let's look at another diet that Dr. Pace is not a big fan of:

HCG Diet

Since we are in the diet section, I have the microphone and we are opening one can of worms after the next, let's talk about the HCG diet. Again, 100 doctors in a room and most likely you would get 50 to love it and 50...not so much! This is the cool part about the relationship with me and Dr. Pace, we can agree to disagree and give you multiple viewpoints on different subjects. Anyway, I tell you all this because if HCG is the route you want to explore, your doctor may agree or disagree.

Let me discuss this for a moment then Dr. Pace will give you his counterpoint, then we will get into his favorite, the keto diet. HCG is human chorionic gonadotropin. HCG is the pregnancy hormone and it basically tells your body to feed from fat, so when eating a low-calorie diet your body uses your fat for fuel instead of going into your muscles for energy. This is the area of controversy - I believe the HCG tells your body to feed off fat, the naysayers believe that just the VLCD is an unsafe way to lose weight. On the website, you will see my tracker. I lost 13 pounds of fat in 50 days. In the HCG world that would be considered a failure. Instead of the 500-calorie diet, I ate calories based on my basal metabolic rate of around 1200 to 1500 calories a day and doing moderate exercise. Did I have my martini? Most nights no, you really want to stay focused during this phase. I would slip a little on the weekends or at social functions, Monday refocused and did OK. Naysayers also say you will lose muscle...hmm...do I look deficient in muscle? So, I am a fan of the HCG diet. We are not going to get into the HCG dosing, protocol, etc. here. If you and your doctor agree, just follow the direction of your doctor. You can also look up the Simeon protocol, the doctor that wrote this in the 1940s. At the time of writing this there are rumors that the FDA is looking at different forms of HCG and further regulations. Check

with us on any updates on social media or check with your
doctor.

Dr. Pace here - thank you Chris and I must admit you did lose
fat and you are looking good. Here is why I don't care about
the HCG diet. I believe it is unsafe and unsustainable for long-
term weight loss. People eat about 500 calories a day but eating so few calories a day is dangerous and puts the body in a
starvation-type state. When the body is starved for calories,
the body's metabolism slows down to preserve energy and in
the long run, that'll sabotage your weight control efforts. The
question is how long someone can sustain a restrictive diet of
500 calories, and the real answer is not long. When a person
gets off the diet, he or she will likely overeat and overindulge
because the body has been in such a restrictive mode. The only
reason why anyone loses weight off this diet is that they're eating 500 calories a day. This directly contradicts what Chris said,
but that's why we are here, to educate, have a friendly debate
and entertain! While calorie intakes are different from person
to person, I say go Keto! Eating 500 calories a day is equiva-
lent to eating one cup of chopped-up chicken breast, with two
servings of fruit and two servings of vegetables — in essence,
it's about the number of calories a person would consume in

just one meal. I think there are more reasonable, sustainable and healthier ways to lose fat. When a body is subsiding off 500 calories a day, the body leeches protein from the muscle in the heart, and that makes the heart muscle irritable, which can lead to ventricular tachycardia and sudden death. That alone makes this cardiologist's heart go into A-fib!! This I know also contradicts Chris' idea of the body feeding off fat. OK - so those are my points and Chris' points. Again, the reason I am writing this book is to educate you, wake you up to different aspects of medicine. "Helping you open your mind, so I won't have to open your heart!" :)

KETO Diet

Dr. Pace here! I have done great on the keto diet! I got wrapped up in life doing many cases in the cardiac unit at the hospital, graduations, steaks, potatoes, red wine, etc. Red wine is my thing as vodka is Chris'. Like we say, everybody has got their thing! 20 pounds snuck up on me! I am guessing that 99% of you have been in the same boat. I went on the keto diet and did well! Just like HCG or any diet, you will have pros and cons. I can hear my colleagues now in the operating room condemning me! Chris agrees with the low carb part and says he eats sort of a WFPB keto diet during his maintenance phase.

let's discuss the keto diet: Low-carb diets have been controversial for decades. Some people assert that these diets raise cholesterol and cause heart disease due to their high-fat content. However, in most scientific studies, low-carb diets prove their worth as healthy and beneficial. Hunger tends to be the worst side effect of dieting. It is one of the main reasons why many people feel miserable and eventually give up. However, low carb eating leads to an automatic reduction in appetite. Studies consistently show that when people cut carbs and eat more protein and fat, they end up eating far fewer calories. I know when I eat a high protein meal, I am less hungry after the meal as opposed to a high carb meal. Cutting carbs is one of the simplest and most effective ways to lose weight. Studies illustrate that people on low-carb diets lose more weight, faster, than those on low-fat diets — even when the latter are actively restricting calories. This is because low-carb diets act to rid excess water from your body, lowering insulin levels and leading to rapid weight loss in the first week or two as was the case with me. Always, always stay hydrated! In studies comparing low-carb and low-fat diets, people restricting their carbs sometimes lose 2–3 times as much weight, without being hungry.

Almost without exception, low-carb diets lead to more short-term weight loss than low-fat diets. Not all fat in your body is the same. Where fat is stored determines how it affects your health and risk of disease. Yes, including cardiovascular disease! The two main types are subcutaneous fat, which is under your skin, and visceral fat, which accumulates in your abdominal cavity and is typical for most overweight men. This is the bad stuff! Visceral fat tends to lodge around your organs. Excess visceral fat is associated with inflammation, insulin resistance, and may drive the metabolic dysfunction so common in my office today! Low-carb diets are very effective at reducing harmful abdominal fat. In fact, a greater proportion of fat that people lose on low-carb diets seems to come from the abdominal cavity which is good. Over time, this should lead to a drastically reduced risk of heart disease and type 2 diabetes and keep you out of my operating room. When you visit your doctor asking about the VDP, more than likely they will mention your cholesterol levels and triglycerides are fat molecules that circulate in your bloodstream. It is well known that high fasting triglycerides — levels in the blood after an overnight fast — are a strong heart disease risk factor. One of the main drivers of elevated triglycerides in sedentary people is carb consumption — especially the simple sugar fructose. Oh boy - don't get Chris started on fruit consumption! Anyway, when people cut carbs, they tend to experience a very dramatic reduction in blood triglycerides - that makes cardiologist happy! On the other hand, low-fat diets often cause triglycerides to increase. High-density lipoprotein (HDL) is often called "good" cholesterol. The higher your levels of HDL relative to "bad" LDL, the lower your risk of heart disease.

Remember, I am here to open your mind, so I don't have to open your heart! One of the best ways to increase "good" HDL levels is to eat fat — and low-carb diets include a lot of fat. Therefore, it is unsurprising that HDL levels increase dramatically on healthy, low-carb diets, while they tend to increase only moderately or even decline on low-fat diets. Low-carb diets tend to be high in fat, which leads to an impressive increase in blood levels of "good" HDL cholesterol. Reduced blood sugar and Insulin levels in low-carb and ketogenic diets can also be particularly helpful for people with diabetes and insulin resistance, which affects millions of people worldwide. Studies prove that cutting carbs lowers both blood sugar and insulin levels drastically. Some people with diabetes who begin a low-carb diet may need to reduce their insulin dosage by 50% almost immediately. In one study in people with type 2 diabetes, 95% had reduced or eliminated their glucose-lowering medication within six months. Please, please - If you take blood sugar medication, talk to your doctor before making changes to your carb intake, as your dosage may need to be adjusted to prevent hypoglycemia. The best way to lower blood sugar and insulin levels are to reduce carb consumption, which may treat and possibly even reverse type 2 diabetes.

Elevated blood pressure, or hypertension, is a significant risk factor for many diseases, including heart disease, stroke and kidney failure. Low-carb diets are an effective way to lower blood pressure, which should reduce your risk of these diseases and help you live longer. Metabolic syndrome is a condition highly associated with your risk of diabetes and heart disease. In fact, metabolic syndrome is a collection of symptoms, which include abdominal obesity, elevated blood pressure, elevated fasting blood sugar levels, high triglycerides, low "good" HDL cholesterol levels. Pretty much Chris' story before, but he never had any sugar issues in his blood. This is also called "syndrome X" in some medical circles. You may hear the term metabolic train wreck here too. Kind of sums up what American physicians see, like 30 times a day! However, a low-carb diet is incredibly effective in treating all five of these symptoms. Under such a diet, these conditions are nearly eliminated. Healthy low-carb diets effectively reverse all five key symptoms of metabolic syndrome. People who have high "bad" LDL are much more likely to have heart attacks. This, in my opinion, is critical to the VDP as we want you healthy on the inside as well as looking good!

I also need to mention C-Reactive Protein or CRP levels and homocysteine here as well. We discussed homocysteine in the B-Vitamins section. While CRP is not part of the core VDP it is an area of cardiology you should be familiar with. In short, it is an inflammatory marker in your blood. A high CRP may or may not be an indication of heart disease. There is also a more specific test that checks a cardiac-specific CRP. I mention this so have a discussion on your CRP level with your doctor. Do some research on these as they are a piece of the puzzle along with LDL.

Let's go back to particle sizes in your cholesterol. Chris had a high VLDL or APOa or very-low-density lipoprotein. The size of the particles is important! Ask your doctor about getting a "fractionation lab panel." Smaller particles are linked to a higher risk of heart disease, while larger particles are linked to a lower risk. It turns out that low-carb diets increase the size of "bad" LDL particles while reducing the number of total LDL particles in your bloodstream. When you eat a low-carb diet, the size of your "bad" LDL particles increases, which reduces their harmful effects.

Let's talk about your brain, glucose, and ketones. Your brain needs glucose, as some parts of it can only burn this type of sugar. That's why your liver produces glucose from protein if you don't eat any carbs. Yet, a large part of your brain can also burn ketones, which are formed during starvation or when carb intake is very low. This is the mechanism behind the ketogenic diet, which has been used for decades to treat epilepsy in children who don't respond to drug treatment. In many cases, this diet can treat children of epilepsy. In one study, over half of the children on a ketogenic diet experienced a greater than 50% reduction in their number of seizures, while 16% became seizure-free. Very low-carb and ketogenic diets are now being studied for other brain conditions as well, including Alzheimer's and Parkinson's disease. What's really cool is these facts combined with the effects of testosterone on the brain. Few things are as well established in nutrition science as the immense health benefits of low-carb and ketogenic diets. As I said, these diets improve your cholesterol, blood pressure and blood sugar, but they also reduce your appetite, boost weight loss and lower your triglycerides. So again, the VDP is not in-tended to be a "diet" per se, but a protocol, a way of life. To sum this up, for the rest of your VDP life, cut or drastically re-duce the carbs in your diet. Chris will cover more of this in the plan at the end of the book. I think we call agree one thing here - cut your carbs!

chapter

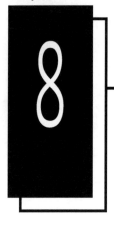

Superfoods

D r. Pace here - I have done a lot of research in this area recently. Again, I received zero hours of nutrition classes in medical school, and agree that super nutrition should be a part of this plan, a high energy smoothie is a way to go. They are easy, affordable and packed with antioxidants. I have done some deep research into omegas, especially when it comes to heart disease.

Yes, you will need a good blender to start. Chris will tell you a story or two, then I will get into some science. I usually make my smoothie when I break my fast after the gym when I feel hungry anytime between about 10 a.m. and noon. This is also when I take my nutraceuticals. It's way cool to think of the hyper nutrition that will hit your body first thing. That is after a ton of water and a great workout. This effectively is my breakfast each day. I start with filtered water, sometimes I may use organic almond milk depending on what phase of the VDP I am in, and if I am restricting calories. Then, I fill it up halfway with either dark cherries, blackberries, raspberries or a blend. Both Dr. Pace and I are big fans of dark cherries. All dark berries have amazing health benefits! Dark cherries are packed with nutrients and rich in antioxidants and anti-inflammatory compounds. They may improve symptoms of arthritis and gout. Dark berries are some of the healthiest foods you can eat, as they are low in calories but high in fiber, vitamin C, and antioxidants. (HCG and Keto friendly) Many berries have proven benefits for heart health. These include lowering blood pressure and cholesterol while reducing oxidative stress.

Chris still here - Let me go off on a little rant here. I think the FDA has its place. I have just seen too much from the inside in my 13 years with big pharma. Let's just say I love dark cherries more than big pharma! What if I told you that the cherry growers were threatened by the FDA? Here is an excerpt from a true story - I can't make this up!!

Otherwise, it said, they could have their products seized or be charged with violating the federal Food, Drug and Cosmetic Act, which defines articles intended to cure, treat or prevent disease. An FDA spokeswoman said the warning was issued after employees in the agency's Detroit office noticed some of the products on the market. The marketing director for the Lansing-based Cherry Marketing Institute said the organization has not been in contact with the FDA about the letters. She said the institute doesn't advise businesses on how to label or describe products. "We're certainly concerned about it and are learning as much as we can," she told the Traverse City Record-Eagle for a story Thursday. "We want these businesses to take the letters seriously and respond to them." The cherry industry has promoted the fruit as a health food in recent years. The marketing institute's Web site carries information on university studies of the fruit's possible health benefits, describing cherries as "a natural pain killer."

Sorry just had to rant a little! Dr. Pace, please talk about some science! Thank you, Chris! First, if you're on the HCG, Keto, or any fat loss diet prescribed by your doctor, please let them know what you're going to include in your smoothie, so as not to cause a problem with your fat loss plan. Case in point, there are some fats here that would be fine on keto, but HCG - not so much. A common thread here will be omega-3 fatty acids. What is omega-3 fatty acid? Also, what is an antioxidant? Omega-3 fatty acids are found in fatty layers of cold-water fish, shellfish, plant and nut oils, English walnuts, flaxseed, algae oils, and fortified foods. You can also get omega-3s as supplements. Food and supplement sources of these fatty acids differ in the forms and amounts they contain.

There are two main types of omega-3 fatty acids: Long-chain omega-3 fatty acids are EPA (eicosapentaenoic acid) and DHA (docosahexaenoic acid). These are plentiful in fish and shellfish. Algae often provide only DHA. Short-chain omega-3 fatty acids are ALA (alpha-linolenic acid). These are found in plants, such as flaxseed. Though beneficial, ALA omega-3 fatty acids have less potent health benefits than EPA and DHA. You'd have to eat a lot to gain the same benefits as you do from fish.

What exactly is an antioxidant? A substance that reduces damage due to oxygen, such as that is caused by free radicals. Think of cells "rusting" as metal does when exposed to oxygen.

Well-known antioxidants include enzymes and other substances, such as vitamin C, vitamin E, and beta carotene, which can counteract the damaging effects of oxidation. Antioxidants are also commonly added to food products such as vegetable oils and prepared foods to prevent or delay their deterioration from the action of air. Antioxidants may possibly reduce the risks of cancer. Antioxidants clearly slow the progression of age-related macular degeneration. Let's continue to what is in Chris' smoothie - You could not fit all this in one serving, so Chris rotates these ingredients each day.

Chia Seeds are full of important nutrients. They are an excellent source of omega-3 fatty acids, rich in antioxidants, and they provide fiber, iron, and calcium. Omega-3 fatty acids help raise HDL cholesterol, the "good" cholesterol that protects against heart attack and stroke.

Hemp Seeds are incredibly nutritious. Hemp seeds contain over 30% fat, not cool on HCG. They are exceptionally rich in two essential fatty acids, linoleic acid (omega-6) and alpha-linolenic acid (omega-3). They also contain gamma-linolenic acid, which has been linked to several health benefits including heart and liver health.

Pumpkin Seeds contain omega-3 and omega-6 fatty acids, antioxidants, and fiber. This combination has benefits for both the heart and liver as well. The fiber in pumpkin seeds helps lower the total amount of cholesterol in the blood and decrease the risk of heart disease.

Cacao Nibs is a highly nutritious chocolate product made from crushed cocoa beans. They're exceptionally rich in antioxidants that help reduce oxidative stress and inflammation. Cocoa Products like cacao nibs have been linked to reduced heart disease and diabetes risk, as well as other health benefits. Keynote - I did not mention milk chocolate here!

Flax Seeds are loaded with nutrients. Flax seeds are high in Omega-3 fats. Flax seeds are a rich source of lignans, which may reduce cancer risk. Flax seeds are rich in dietary fiber. Flax seeds may improve cholesterol and help lower blood pressure.

Turmeric contains bioactive compounds with powerful medicinal properties. Curcumin is the compound in turmeric and is a natural anti-inflammatory compound turmeric dramatically increases the antioxidant capacity of the body. Curcumin boosts brain-derived neurotrophic factor linked to improved brain function and a lower risk of brain diseases. There is impressive data with pancreatic cancer as well. A little downfall here with the Turmeric, it is truly an amazing substance, it is an acquired taste though as it can really throw off your smoothie taste.

Vegan **protein powder,** again this could be an entire book on protein powders. Note I put protein powder in bold and not vegan. Seems like whey protein is the thing to do but keep in mind it is derived from a cow that Chris is not a huge fan of. Get with your doctor on the right ingredients in your protein powder. These are nice for recovery after a workout. Some say protein before a workout, again, could be another book.

These smoothies are quick and easy to incorporate into your diet. They are available everywhere, in malls, etc. You can go crazy with kale, bananas, spinach, etc. I am also a big fan of juicing as well. This is simply extracting the juice from fruits and vegetables using a juicer or extractor. Powerful condensed nutrients! Celery, apple, kale, and wheatgrass is a favorite. We could write another book or chapter on superfoods. Just find one that works for you and keep your doctor up to date, so let's move on to the plan!

The Plan

9

I am going to hand this over to Chris and I will chime in at the end. Chris has lived this more than I and he has some tricks and can discuss the financial aspects of all this as well. Thank you, Dr. Pace! Hopefully, by now you have feelings of excitement. I know when I first discovered all of this in the VDP, I could not wait to get started. I remember the first 3 weeks after my first insertion, were the longest three weeks of my life, in a good way. Kind of like mid- December for a child waiting for Christmas. I had discovered hormones before peptides, and I had the same emotions after starting my first round of peptides. I say all of this because the first part of the plan it's to make sure your mind is in the right place. If you have emotions of skepticism and questions that is understandable, but this process will be a lot better if you have emotions of excitement as I did.

Close your eyes and visualize yourself thin, in shape, or muscular. If you can visualize it and see it in your mind, I am sure you can achieve it. I am sure you were like me, tried everything in the world, many failures, therefore your mind may not be in the right place. You will have many temptations along the way. I just thought back to a graduation dinner for my daughter at Maggiano's. Pasta, bread, and the wine were flowing as I sat with my salad with balsamic vinaigrette. The martini did taste good though, and I kept my paws out of the breadbasket! I tell you that quick story because you will have temptations, and again it just turns into a mindset and commitment.

Another quick story is the reward in the satisfaction you get from the VDP. I was on a little vacation with my daughter at Deerfield Beach, FL right after my round of HCG. Before this if I was at the beach, I would wait till I was close to the water layout my towel, take off my shirt and head straight into the water. The goal would be to minimize the exposure of my roundness to the world. For the first time in I don't know how many years I left the hotel and walked three blocks to the beach with my shirt off. Just that feeling alone just brought feelings of amazement, confidence, it was almost like a reward to myself. Shortly thereafter, people start noticing the weight loss and that is a great feeling as well. Ok - so what is the plan you ask?

Before we go any further, let's answer the question of how much all this costs? The short answer is between $30 and $300 a month. While there is no concrete VDP program for everyone, therefore there is not one cost for everyone. First, find a clinic and get a blood test. This should be easy to find on our website or you can check with your current doctor. Prices for this are all over the board. Some clinics charge for the consult, some not. Your insurance may or may not pay for the consult and the blood test. Just ask the clinic the cash price for these items beforehand.

Now that you have your blood test results, your doctor will compare these to how you are feeling and review with you. Many medical assistants and nurses in offices are good at these conversations as they have had special training in this area. After that conversation, you will have a clinical plan concerning the VDP. My progression through the VDP has been

137

like the chapters of this book in a chronological perspective. After your consult and lab review you will have your plan with dates and goals. The last pages of this book are designed for this conversation with your doctor.

Let's get back to the financial aspects of the VDP. I will break it down for you. Like I said, this could cost you only $30 a month. You may just need thyroid medication; your other hormone levels are good, and you follow a good keto diet and do some HIIRT and you are good to go. Also, you may be on a tight budget, working overtime, raising kids, paying a mortgage, I get it for sure! In 2008 I was one of those guys you read about, lost it all! I am not coming to you from an ivory tower here. You may be killing it in your career, a stay at home mom married to a doctor or Hollywood actor. The point here is the VDP can be individualized to your needs and your financial situation. The two biggest upfront expenses here will be the BHRT and the peptides. The BHRT can be around $100 a month for females and around $150 per month for males. Men require about 10x the amount of testosterone as females and the manufacturing process for good, pure pharmaceutical grade pellets can be expensive. Peptides are all over the board, so I hesitate to throw out a number here. Just ask your clinic about their prices. You may want to do one round of BHRT first to see how you feel, then add on peptides the second round. Again, listen to your doctor and your wallet. HIIRT can be free outside on your own, or you could join a class and would be the price of a high-end gym membership. Keto grocery bill can be a little high as it is high protein. HCG could get expensive, but you have a lower grocery bill and it is temporary. While you are on any of the fat loss phases, you should not see a restaurant bill, or the inside of a restaurant unless you are working in one. For the nutra-ceuticals, if you are on BHRT you can start with the DIM. I have heard of clinics bundling a few of the nutras to get you start-ed. Again, listen to your doctor and your wallet. Superfoods smoothie on an individual serving is not expensive if made at home. The initial shock maybe buying all the ingredients at once. To start, just get a frozen bag of berries and some chia seeds. As you move along, you can buy a bag of cacao nibs, then some flax, etc. A jug of powdered protein is about $25.

So that was for the 98% of you. The hard working, kid raising bill paying person out there. Now I will address the well healed. Nothing wrong with a little success, I can appreciate that. So, you have read this, your excited, your sleeves are rolled up and you are ready to dive in. In that case, get your blood test and get on BHRT yesterday if you and your doctor agree. You should leave the office with all your nutras that day. Find a good HIIRT class in your area. Get on the best diet for you. At your 4-6 week follow up visit with your doctor, have a peptide discussion and get on the best peptide for your situation. Go to the store and buy your ingredients for your smoothie. Enjoy!

To review, hopefully there will be bits and pieces of the VDP that work for all of you. It is truly an amazing journey and I cannot think of a better investment than your health. Keep in touch and let us know your progress and please share any pearls you may have.

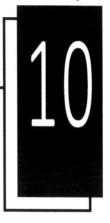

Infrared Sauna/ Laser

Hi! Dr. Pace here. You are saying, wait. the book is over, I got this! I have the plan and I am off to my doctor. Well, Chris and I were in the Cath lab talking about his success and the topic of saunas came up. I shared with Chris that the VDP is all about transforming yourself and making you healthy, and there are a lot of aspects about longevity or as some anti-aging in the VDP. I shared some data I came across concerning Finnish, or people in Finland. In most Finland homes, they have dry infrared saunas and have a longer life span. I will share some of that data in a second. Chris was interested but his remark was that it would not be feasible to include sauna therapy in the VDP, because quite simply we do not have saunas in our houses of which

I understood. Have I mentioned that Chris is kind of a freak? A week later I get a text of a picture of Chris sweating in a sauna. The message was "look what I found on Facebook for $500". We decided that in the spirit of transparency we would tell that story. I also do believe wholeheartedly in this therapy for longevity and cardiovascular health. I do realize we have limited access to saunas, therefore not part of the core VDP.

Let me share some data from a study out of Finland concerning the longevity of the Finnish people, then Chris will share his experience with one of those fat loss lasers. Researchers from the University of Eastern

Finland tracked 2,300 middle-aged men for an average of 20 years. They categorized the men into three groups according to how often they used a sauna each week. The men spent an average of 14 minutes per visit baking at 175° F heat. Chris does 20 minutes at 135 degrees. Over the course of the study, 49% of men who went to a sauna once a week died, compared with 38% of those who went two to three times a week, and just 31% of those who went four to seven times a week. Frequent visits to a sauna were also associated with lower death rates from cardiovascular disease and stroke. Chris is in his sauna 4 to 7 times a week!

Thank you, Dr. Pace! Yes, I love the sauna! One more quick note and we are done. We mention the laser because in many of the clinics you may see these sculpting lasers. We decided not to include this in the core VDP like saunas just due to access and quite honestly, it would not be in my budget. I had been curious about these, but I always had too much fat to lose before I could even qualify for the therapy. I also saw the freezing sculpting and the heating sculpting. I was able to strike up a deal with a heating sculpting laser. In complete honesty and transparency, I cannot give an honest assessment due to the timing of publishing this book and my treatments. I am currently doing these weekly sessions and will let you know my findings on YouTube or Instagram soon. Again, just keeping everything in the VDP and my journey transparent.

Chris and I want to thank you sincerely for joining us on this journey! My dream is that this is the start of a platform that will help people achieve their goals and live a healthy long life. I have big plans for volume 2 and have started collecting manuscripts from my colleagues and it is looking exciting! I hope to meet you in person one day and please share your success with us on social media!

Now some before and after pictures of Chris.

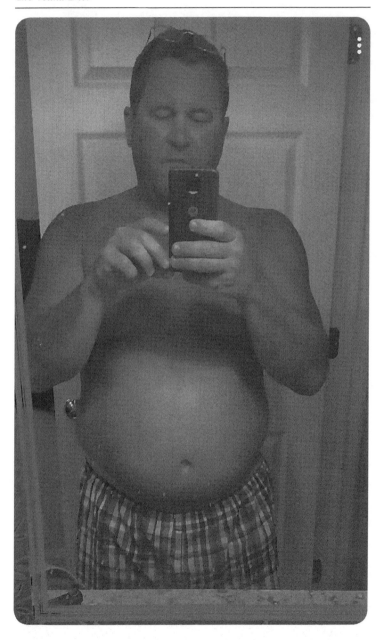

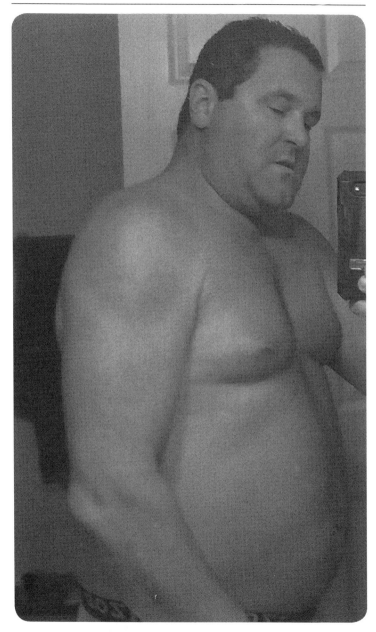

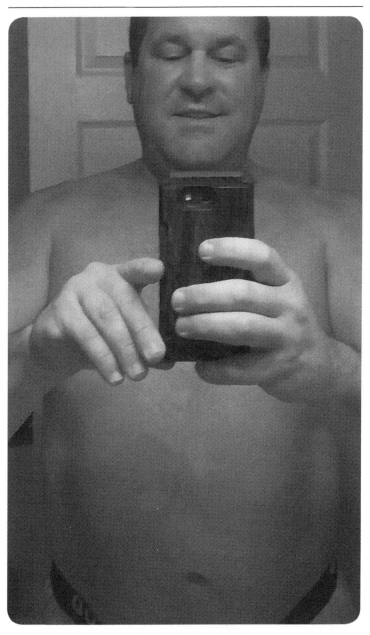

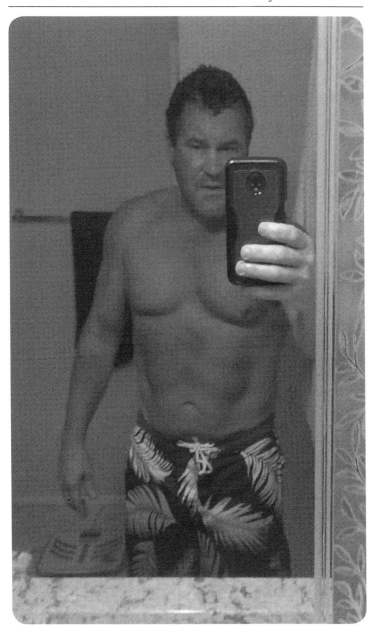

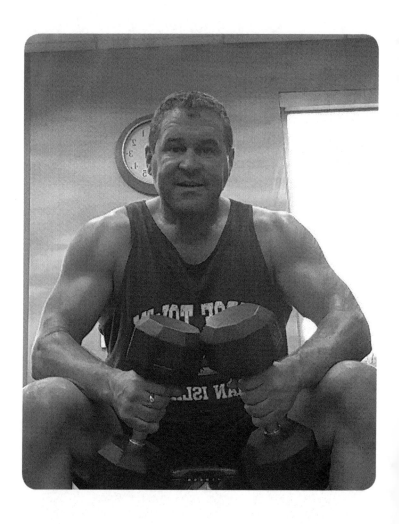

Made in the USA
Columbia, SC
31 July 2020

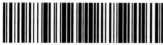

14069440R00083